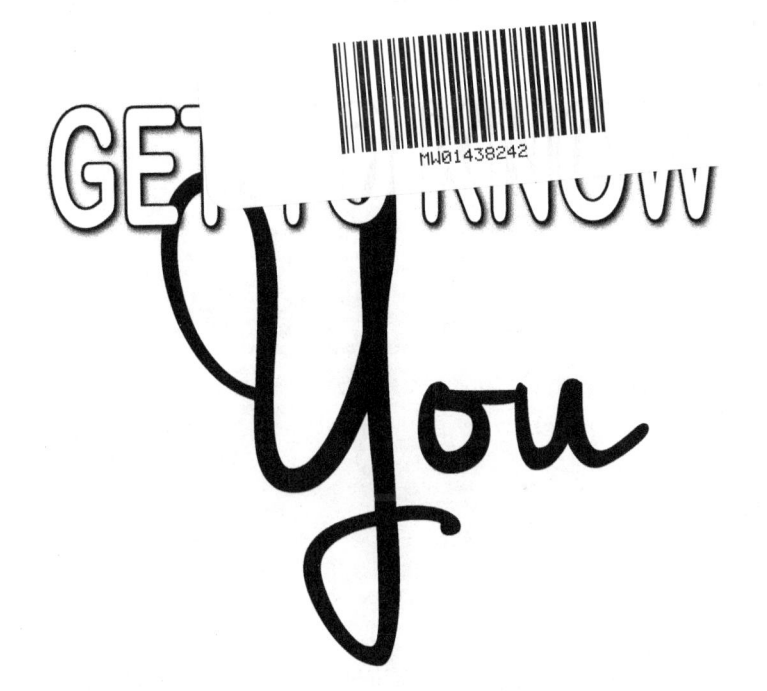

GET TO KNOW You

Jodi Reeves

Get To Know You
© Jodi Reeves 2019

All rights reserved. No part of this publication may be reproduced, stored in a retrieval system, or transmitted in any form or by any means, electronic, mechanical, photocopying, recording or otherwise, without the prior written permission of the author.

ISBN: 978-1-925833-41-6 (Paperback)
978-1-925833-42-3 (eBook)

A catalogue record for this book is available from the National Library of Australia

Printed in China by Ocean Reeve Publishing
www.oceanreevepublishing.com
Published by Jodi Reeves and Ocean Reeve Publishing
www.jodi-reeves.com

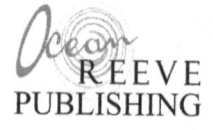

Ocean REEVE PUBLISHING

Contents

Question 1	What is your favourite colour?	3
Question 2	What is your favourite smell?	5
Question 3	What is your favourite season?	7
Question 4	What is your favourite TV show?	9
Question 5	What is your favourite piece of clothing?	13
Question 6	What is your favourite book?	15
Question 7	What is your favourite movie?	17
Question 8	What is your favourite song?	19
Question 9	Who is your favourite artist?	21
Question 10	Who is your favourite musician?	23
Question 11	What is your favourite car?	25
Question 12	Where is your favourite holiday destination?	27
Question 13	What is your favourite meal?	29
Question 14	What is your all-time favourite food?	31
Question 15	Who is your favourite actor?	35
Question 16	What is your favourite sound?	37
Question 17	What is your favourite emotion?	39
Question 18	Who is your favourite politician or political figure?	45
Question 19	Who was/is your favourite teacher?	47
Question 20	What is your favourite drink?	49
Question 21	What is your favourite animal?	51
Question 22	What is your favourite flower?	53
Question 23	What is your favourite tree?	55
Question 24	What is your favourite gift to receive?	57
Question 25	What is your favourite gift to give?	59
Question 26	What was your favourite birthday/birthday celebration?	61
Question 27	What is your favourite thing to cook?	63
Question 28	Who is your favourite author?	65

Question 29	What is your favourite exercise?	67
Question 30	What is your favourite pen to write with?	69
Question 31	What is your favourite metal?	71
Question 32	What is your favourite crystal?	73
Question 33	What is your favourite activity/hobby?	75
Question 34	What is your favourite sport?	77
Question 35	What is your favourite subject?	79
Question 36	What is your favourite herb?	81
Question 37	What is your favourite shell?	83
Question 38	What makes you smile?	85
Question 39	What makes you laugh?	87
Question 40	What makes you cry?	89
Question 41	What makes you scared?	91
Question 42	What makes you jump for joy?	93
Question 43	What makes you retreat?	99
Question 44	What makes you hide?	101
Question 45	What makes you dance?	103
Question 46	What are you hiding?	105
Question 47	What makes you reflect?	107
Question 48	What makes you feel confident?	109
Question 49	What makes you doubt yourself?	111
Question 50	What gets you talking?	113
Question 51	What is your favourite personal attribute?	115
Question 52	As a child what did you dream of being when you grew up?	117
Question 53	What do you feel is your weakness?	119
Question 54	What do you, or could you do, to overcome your weakness?	121
Question 55	What inspires, drives or motivates you?	123
Question 56	What holds you back?	125
Question 57	Who supports you?	127
Question 58	Who helps bring out the best in you?	129
Question 59	Who challenges you?	131

Question 60	Who teaches you the most?	133
Question 61	How do you best learn?	135
Question 62	What do you 'beat' yourself up about?	137
Question 63	What was a major turning point in your life?	139
Question 64	Do you like tea or coffee, mugs or cups, tea bags or teapot, instant or ground?	141
Question 65	Where is your dream location to live?	143
Question 66	What is your biggest success to date?	145
Question 67	What is your biggest mistake?	147
Question 68	What do you doubt?	149
Question 69	What do you trust?	151
Question 70	What don't you trust?	153
Question 71	What excuse do you use most often?	155
Question 72	What is your driving or primary intention?	157
Question 73	What or who encourages you to be the best you?	159
Question 74	Who do you love?	161
Question 75	What do you love?	163
Question 76	Who do you admire?	165
Question 77	What traits do you respect in others?	167
Question 78	Who would you like to be like?	169
Question 79	What do you most like to talk about?	171
Question 80	What can't you do?	173
Question 81	What can't you live without?	175
Question 82	What do you wish you did better?	177
Question 83	What does strength look, feel or sound like to you?	179
Question 84	What does weakness look, feel or sound like to you?	181
Question 85	Whose voice do you hear in your head?	183
Question 86	What achievement are you most proud of?	187

Question 87	Do you believe in fairies or magic?	**189**
Question 88	What do you dislike about yourself?	**191**
Question 89	What does God mean to you?	**193**
Question 90	What makes you nervous?	**195**
Question 91	What makes you feel helpless?	**197**
Question 92	What makes you feel capable?	**199**
Question 93	What do you know to be true?	**201**
Question 94	What do you believe in?	**203**
Question 95	What do you dream about?	**205**
Question 96	What does paradise mean to you?	**207**
Question 97	Why do you think you are here, at this time, in this place, with the people who surround you?	**209**
Question 98	What are your favourite memories and experiences in your life so far?	**211**
Question 99	What negative stories do you tell yourself about yourself, your past, your abilities or your future?	**215**
Question 100	Who are you?	**217**
Question 101	Who do you wish to be? What can you do right now to become, or move closer to being, exactly who you wish to be?	**221**

Acknowledgements

There are a few people who I have to thank for their support, love, input and presence in my life. Without them, I don't think I would be standing here holding my first book in my hands.

My parents; you have always supported me and given me the best you possibly could. You instilled in me a belief that anything is possible and even if I doubted that many times over the years, the belief that I could do and be anything was still there, quietly assuring me.

To every client, and every follower I have had, thank you. Thank you for trusting me and allowing me to share my ideas, thoughts and wisdom with you. Always remember, from your authentic vulnerability your unique light shines.

To Ocean, your wisdom, knowledge and support has guided me through this process, but there is more than that. I will never forget the fear and nerves I had as I sat across from you in a coffee shop and first shared my dream for this book with you. A dream that had safely and comfortably sat inside of me for so many years. It felt like a make-or-break moment for me and I felt so vulnerable. Your genuine response of, "This is such an original concept and so many people in the world need this book; it will have a big impact on the lives of many people," is what allowed this dream—my dream—to be realised. Regardless of what happens from here, I will never forget your encouragement. Superman really does suit you!

Jason, The Flash, what an incredible and patient person you are. Yes, you are professional, but more than that, you are caring and so supportive of an individual's creative expression. I know this book and this author haven't been the easiest, and without you, I am not sure I would have got to this point of actually holding a book—my book—in my hands. You help dreams come true.

To my children, Madi, Mitch, Lillee and Lexi, you have watched me grow, change and shine, but you have also witnessed me stopping and crumbling in self-doubt – more than once. You forever encourage me and tell me I am capable of great things, even though it should be my job to tell you that. You are one of the huge reasons I do this. My darlings, please know you can follow your dreams, and it is never too late!

Most importantly to my husband, James. You have held the vision of who I can be and what I can do and achieve for so many years. You held that vision for me when I just couldn't see it, and you held firm in your belief that I am capable of almost anything. You work tirelessly to support our whole family, but specifically, my dreams. You have never given up on me when I wavered, stopped or sat in procrastination for years, you just lovingly encouraged me to move forward and to finally live my dreams!

And to you, if you are holding this book in your hands, I thank you. I wish I could jump out of the pages and hug you for valuing my vision enough to buy and read my book. I wish you nothing but joy and happiness, and I hope you go out and chase your own dreams.

Preface

Are you struggling with relationships, or money, or your weight, or your health or even just life?

Have you read *The Secret* or taken manifestation classes and, if so, have you or are you practising what they suggest, yet nothing seems to be manifesting or shifting in your life as you would like?

Do you feel misunderstood by others?
Do you struggle to identify your 'path', your 'purpose'?
Do you feel left out or left behind?
Do you sometimes just feel lost?
Do you feel something is missing in your life but you can't quite pin point or identify what?
Do you spend time getting to know other people, yet you don't really know yourself?
Do you feel forgotten, ignored or not valued by others?
Do you sometimes 'be' the person you think others want you to be not the person you truly are?
Do you know who you are?

This, I believe, is often the vital missing piece!!!

I struggled with all of the above. One random day, thanks to a conversation with my then fourteen-year-old son, I realised or finally admitted that I didn't know me!!

I was a people-pleaser; I was always trying to please others. In fact I had become obsessed with trying to please everyone else. I had listened to the opinions of other people and put others and their needs or even their wants ahead of my own for so long that I had actually forgotten not just what I wanted but who I even was. I no longer knew what I liked and often even what I believed! As much as I loved being a wife and a mother, I had also allowed myself to get lost in those roles.

My son stopped me one day out of the blue and said, "Mum, what makes you happy? What do you like? What would you like to do?"

I couldn't answer him so I brushed him off but he wouldn't have it.

He said, "Okay then, what is your favourite TV show? What is your favourite meal?"

I couldn't even answer these basic questions. His response shocked me ... "Well Mum," he said seriously as he looked me square in the eyes, "until you know yourself, you are no good to us."

It was then, right in that moment, that I realised I didn't know myself and that knowing myself mattered. It mattered to me, it mattered to my kids, it mattered to my husband, it mattered to my health, it mattered to my relationships, it mattered to any potential business, and it mattered to my future.

It mattered!!!

In nurturing others' and my relationships with other people and trying for so long to do the 'right' thing, whatever that may have been, I had forgotten about me. I had ignored my wants and desires in the pursuit of discovering and meeting other people's needs, wants and desires.

I had become so concerned about what other people thought, that I forgot what I thought. I even forgot to care what I thought.

I so wanted to be liked and accepted by others that I forgot to make sure I liked myself first!

I realised, in that moment, that the key to what was missing in my life, the reason I struggled with direction in my life, the reason I felt unfulfilled and I couldn't identify what my passions were, was because I had no relationship with the most important person in my life ... ME!!!

How do we do this? How did we get here? Where or how do we lose sight of who we are? When and how do we forget what we like?

The answer is simple.

We focus more on others than we do on ourselves.

For me, I focussed on being the best mother and wife I could be. As I found my feet as a mother I also desperately wanted other people to 'like' me, to validate me. I wanted to be seen and heard and valued because deep down I didn't value my contribution. I felt I had to make myself worthy of being born. I spent more time worrying and wondering what other people thought, and less and less time wondering or caring what I thought or wanted. I ignored me and focussed most, if not all, of my attention outwards. I focussed on other people and what I thought they thought, what I thought they wanted, what I thought they felt, what I thought they said, what I thought they meant, what I thought they liked.

By doing this, and for the most part ignoring or not even considering what I thought, wanted, felt, or liked, I ignored me and in turn my relationship with self. I lost touch with me.

I slowly but surely lost contact with who I was. It was gradual; I didn't notice it at the time but I felt it. I just didn't know exactly what I was feeling or what to do about it, so I kept going. I kept focussing on and trying to please other people.

Surely if I just keep focussing on other people and what they want, and try and meet those needs, I will be happy … and I will be liked … and I will be valued … and I will be heard … and I will be seen!

Surely!

No, it doesn't work that way. In doing this, I lost myself. I forgot who I was and my relationship with me slowly diminished over time. I ignored the most important person in my life, ME, and my relationship with self suffered because of my choices.

What we think, what we do, what we focus on, what we give mental and emotional time to builds our neurological pathways or circuits. Now I am not a scientist or neurological expert, but here it is explained very simply: our neurological pathways, which we create through repetition, become our subconscious defaults for thoughts, actions and even at times emotions. These pathways are our brain's way of quickly sorting through the thousands of messages received through our senses every minute. Instead of having to consider and assess each stimulus or message, our mind goes down the most 'used' neurological pathway.

So when I thought something as simple as *what will we have for dinner?* My mind could go easily to *what would my children or husband like that meal to be?* But it wouldn't naturally go to what I might want that meal to be, as that pathway was very weak. The neurological pathway to my desire was like a path through a thick forest with long grass and trees. A path that had only been walked on once or twice. Yet the pathway to what my children or family might want was like a three-lane highway – well-established and easy to fly along without conscious thought.

This was reinforced by my desire to be a good mother, to live up to society's expectations, to never be seen as selfish and my very well-learned habit of always putting others first. All well-intentioned desires, perhaps even admirable intentions, but this focus left me unsure of who I was and with no idea that this disconnection with self was a greater problem.

The neurological pathway that connected me with me was weak. I don't think that pathway can be completely broken but it was very weak. My brain, through the neural circuits that I had exercised most often, those that linked me to other people and their needs and desires, automatically ensured I thought more about others than I thought about myself and I knew more about others than I knew of myself. I had inadvertently 'wired' myself to think about everyone else before I thought about me.

Many of us take time to get to know other people; we even pride ourselves on it, and in the process we can forget who we are ourselves. We work the neurological pathways that connect us to what other people want or need or feel or desire but we allow the neurological pathways that connect us to what we want or need or feel or desire to become dormant, stagnant; it is like that pathway goes into atrophy. All while the neurons firing to ensure we think about other people are getting the best workout ever, and thanks to this they are kept strong and over time get even stronger!

I realised this had to change. I had to get to know me! And I had to get to know me first, before I worked on my relationships with others, or a business, or my purpose, or manifestation, or anything else. The first step was working on getting to know me. I needed to rediscover who Jodi Reeves was. I needed to rebuild my neural pathways to my own desires, to my own needs, to me.

But how? How could I do this?

Now that I knew the problem, I felt like this was the missing piece; but I was faced with a new problem. What did I need to do about it? How could I fix it?

When I first started asking myself questions and trying to 'get to know me', it was actually shocking and even embarrassing how little I knew about myself. But through a series of questions, some really basic and others a little more involved and personal, I began to understand who Jodi was again. I also realised that this was going to be an ongoing process, as we change so often. You don't get to know yourself once and the work is done; we need to stay in touch with ourselves and continue to nurture that relationship. We need to continue to 'fire' or exercise that neural pathway.

I admit I still struggle with this at times but I now refuse to hide. I refuse to hide from myself, from others, and I don't ignore the importance of my relationship with me. I have learned (okay, I am still learning) to put myself first. I have accepted that this isn't a bad thing; this doesn't mean I am egotistical or 'up myself' as the teenage me would worry about. I don't do this at the expense of others; in fact quite the opposite. When I nurture myself, and know who I am, those around me get to experience a much better version of me and what I give, emotionally and of my time, I give freely.

During this process of self-discovery or, more accurately, rediscovery I was 'gifted' 101 questions that can help us build the connection to self, to re-fire the neural pathway to YOU, and I have found these questions to be one of the most powerful and positive tools we can use to get to know ourselves, to reignite those neural connections.

In this book, you will be asked 101 questions. I recommend you answer one question a day for 101 days. Some questions you may answer easily, others may require a bit more thought. To be honest, for me, most have taken quite a lot of thought. That is how disconnected from self I was, how atrophied my neural pathways were; yet through these questions I have reconnected and continue to connect with myself.

The big thing here is honesty. What do YOU truly like or feel or desire or experience? This is about YOU!! This is about getting to know the incredible, unique person you are and sometimes it is about acknowledging how little you currently know about your current self.

In these five or ten minutes a day, you are to think of no one other than yourself!

Some questions are accompanied by an activity, others by a quote or insight regarding this practice. Doing these extras alongside the questions will strengthen the process. Sit in the presence or awareness of the question, your answer, and the accompanying information.

All relationships require work and the relationship with self is no different. The following 101 questions and accompanying activities, quotes, affirmations or thoughts are a fun and simple way to work on your relationship with you … to build and nurture your sacred relationship with self.

You may choose to answer these questions out loud or in your head. I like to grab a journal and record each answer, with the day's date. I have been through these questions three times now and I know I will revisit them many more times.

Life can distract us at times, responsibilities can overwhelm us and we can feel the disconnect happening. When this occurs, I come back to this process. It is interesting to look back over my past answers and see which ones stay the same and which ones change. My answer to the first question, a simple question that you would think never changes, has changed each time.

We grow, we evolve and we change and through these changes we can forget who we are again. Get to Know You will always bring you back to you.

Welcome to the journey back to self.

Know you
Be you
Love you
Live Life Fulfilled

Much Love
Jodi xxxx

"Someone will always be prettier. Someone will always be smarter. Someone will always be younger. But they will never be you."

— **Kayne West**

Royal Blue

Question 1
What is your favourite colour?

As you go to sleep tonight take three deep breaths and imagine yourself breathing in your favourite colour.

Allow the colour to fill your body from the tips of your toes to the top of your head. Then imagine the colour radiating out from around you.

As you do this, you can ask when and how you can use your special colour. Surround yourself in the beautiful colour that is your favourite as you drift off to sleep.

Colours can deliver messages, so ask your colour if it has a message for you. Listen to these messages.

You can use this meditation anytime you feel a bit disconnected from self or even if you struggle with any of the questions over the next 101 days.

Look at ways to build your favourite colour into your life.

That might be in a bunch of flowers or the clothes you wear, or your bed linen, or the notebook you journal in, or a candle you burn. These are simple yet powerful ways to include your favourite colour in your day.

"The most courageous act is still to think for yourself."

– Coco Chanel

Question 2
What is your favourite smell?

Many of us don't think of our sense of smell as often as we do our other senses, yet it is a powerful sense, which has the ability to trigger memories and emotions.

Tonight, sit quietly and take three deep breaths.

Imagine and focus on the smell you identified today as your favourite.

As you breathe, imagine that smell, smell it all around you.

How does your smell make you feel?

Content   Beautiful
Secure   Happy
Hopeful   Strong
Renewed   Successful

What positive emotion do you feel, as you smell your favourite smell?

GET TO KNOW YOU

Remember that feeling, embrace it, and acknowledge it.

If you ever are in a situation where you would like to feel that emotion but you are struggling to feel it, you can smell 'your' smell and you will feel that emotion. This smell has the power to create an instant change in your 'state', in the way you feel.

Thank your body for the ability to smell such beautiful smells.

What can you do to ensure you have regular access to some of your favourite smells?

We can imagine or remember a smell, recreating it in our mind and imagination, but to actually smell the smell is powerful.

Question 3

What is your favourite season?

Did you know you can use your favourite season to increase your productivity across the entire year?

There is a belief, and for the most part it is a solid one, that spring, for example, is the time to start new projects, to clarify your purpose, and plan your year. To sow the seeds for your coming year's work so to speak.

Similarly, winter is thought to be a time of reflection, hibernation almost, quiet yet purposeful planning, regrouping.

Energetically, each season aligns with stages of growth and activity. Much like it does in the plant and animal worlds.

Here, though, is the difference:

Not all people are the same, just like not all plants are the same. If you were a Jonquil or a Geranium, winter is your time to bloom, your time to shine and summer will be your time of hibernation. If you happen to be a Snapdragon, autumn would be your season of glory.

Just like those flowers you may find your season for emergence and activity is in fact winter.

Pay attention to the feelings each season triggers in you. Some people have far more energy in winter, others in summer or autumn or spring.

Your 'favourite' season will probably also be your most productive season; this is the season to identify your goals for the year. Your plans will have more power; it is the time to sow your seeds and get things started.

The thoughts, ideas and activities that you plant in your favourite season will have the best chance of success.

Your favourite season will give you the ability to set up your year with more ease than at other times. You will feel more in alignment and in the flow during 'your' season.

Use the seasons and the energy of the season to more easily step into your own greatness!

Question 4
What is your favourite TV show?

The TV shows we watch can be really important in our lives. I have never really given it too much thought and when I was given today's question, I just thought it was a bit of fun.

As I have said, my son instigated this process when he asked me various questions about me that I couldn't answer. And I didn't just not know the answer; I was incredibly uncomfortable even thinking about it!

Like many teenagers he watched a lot of TV; in fact he would devour a whole series. Anything from *The Brady Bunch* to *Hamish and Andy*, he would just watch them for hours and like many parents I would become concerned about his TV habits … was he watching too much? I often talked to him, explaining that I felt he should watch less TV. He would never argue but nothing changed and one day, fuelled by my own fear and judgement, I got angry with him about it. Here is how he responded. I remember three specific series he referred to:

"Mum do you know why I watch all these shows? Most of the time I am not watching them mindlessly; I am watching them deliberately. I pick the shows I need at different times.

I watch *Seinfeld* on the days that everything has gone wrong and I feel like I am bursting inside and wish I could punch someone. It makes me laugh and it changes my focus. I can even sometimes laugh about what has happened in my day.

I watch *Friends* because it gives me hope that one day I will have good friends. They are all different but they support each other and are there for each other. Maybe that will happen for me one day.

I watch *Bewitched* because it makes me think anything is possible, that one day things might just magically change.

These aren't just TV shows, Mum, they are how I cope. Not by ignoring what is happening, but by seeing it can one day be different. When I get home from a day at school I need a way to change how I am feeling, and these shows do that."

Now obviously I don't recall word for word what he said but I will never forget the conversation.

This question reminded me that this can be the power of TV shows. Sometimes they are just for entertainment but we can use them to change our thinking, change our energy and shift our perspective!

I know the 'home' type shows helped me dream again. During a very challenging financial time I felt like

I lost the right to dream, these shows helped me get it back! And when I need a laugh, to change my negative state, *The Big Bang Theory* never fails me.

TV shows can be powerful.

Pay attention to how you 'feel' when you watch certain shows, your favourite shows. You may be able to use them more purposefully in your life!

"Authenticity. The courage to be yourself."

– Anonymous

Question 5
What is your favourite piece of clothing?

I don't think it is so important how clothes make us look to the outside world, but I do believe it is very important how our clothes make us feel. It is not important what others think but it is very important what we think.

Feeling good about what you wear will affect your energy and the energy you put out into the universe, the energy that walks with you and greatly influences your focus and experiences. You can pretend it doesn't; you can pretend you like things you don't but your energy will emit the truth.

Knowing what you like to wear, knowing what makes you feel best, is a part of self-connection, self-awareness and self-projection.

Acknowledging what you like to wear, why you like it, how it makes you feel can help you harness the power of clothes.

Yes, they have power.

If you like jeans, have the best possible jeans you can; if you like long flowing dresses, go and buy yourself a new one; if you love track pants, treat yourself to a new pair in a colour you love. Wear gorgeous underwear, just for you; buy new socks and then feel good and worthy and special as you wear them!

You don't have to spend a lot, although you can if you want to. If you can't buy anything right now, just go and start looking. See what you like; look at what you like; touch the fabrics; try on new styles; soak in the colours! Pull your wardrobe apart and see what is actually in there; you might be surprised.

Clothes can, will, and do affect you; they can affect your energy and your feelings, and you can make sure the effect is as positive as possible, allowing you to step into the world feeling your best YOU!! I don't care if that is in a tracksuit or a cocktail dress, as long as you truly feel good!

Do it for YOU! Dress for you. Dress to feel the best 'you' possible.

Question 6
What is your favourite book?

Books are one of our greatest teachers, our easiest escapes and our most loyal entertainers.

What do you love about your favourite book?
How does it make you feel?
What does it teach you?
What dreams does it trigger within you?

You may have chosen a book you recall from your childhood. Is it the book you love or the person who used to read it to you?

Do you love the book because it entertained you, amused you, taught you, or does it allow you to escape within its pages?

It may be the characters. What do these characters stir within you? How do you identify with them?

It may be the story. What does the story show you, teach you, remind you of, or how does it align with yours?

Books can influence us in many ways: they can trigger memories, help us identify what is important to us, teach us, enlighten us, identify what we miss, or desire, or enjoy, or perhaps return us to a part of our past we haven't been acknowledging. A book can stir emotions and feelings.

What is it you love and remember about your favourite book?

Question 7
What is your favourite movie?

Movies have the ability to transport us. They can transport us to a different time, a different world and different realities.

Much like your favourite book, you may love your favourite movie because of the feelings it evoked within you, or the potential it showed you, or the journey it took you on, or the message it delivered.

It may be the memories of that time of your life when you first watched the movie, or it may be that it triggered emotions within you, or took you on a journey for a while, away from where you were.

What is it that you love about your favourite movie?
Is it the way it makes you feel, or the memories it stirs within you?

GET TO KNOW YOU

Go and re-watch your favourite movie and allow yourself to feel. To feel whatever it is that it triggers within you.

What journey does it take you on?

Question 8
What is your favourite song?

Do you sometimes hear the advice, "Focus on increasing or raising your vibration", and do you ever think, "How do I do that?"

One powerful and easy way is to listen to music, and more specifically your favourite music.

Pay attention to how your favourite music makes you feel. You can then consciously use it to increase your energy, improve your positivity, change your current feeling, increase your productivity, overcome your procrastination, strengthen your connection to self, or to motivate you when needed.

The list is endless.

Everyone would benefit from a playlist of their favourite songs. Pressing 'play' on that playlist when feeling less than ideal can be truly powerful and can facilitate important energetic shifts within us.

Do you use music to your advantage?

You should! Music can be far more than just entertainment ... far more!

Question 9
Who is your favourite artist?

Art, great art, helps us feel, provokes us to feel, and encourages us to feel. It can help us access emotions we have often buried or ignored ... if we give it permission, it can do all of this.

Artists can transport us with a mere brush stroke or the feathering of a pencil or the blending of colours or the timing of a shutter. Their vision on canvas or paper, or clay can leave an impression far beyond the physical. We can be transported by their medium to places and times long gone or not yet experienced, to emotions long buried or denied, to dreams we haven't yet had the courage to dream.

Great art is not determined merely by its technical components. It is determined by its uncanny ability to transport, transform, touch and move us. Great artists share with us a part of their being, their energy and impact us with more than their artistic ability; they touch us with their soul and they often leave us forever changed.

"I've always loved the idea of not being what people expect me to be."

— **Dita Von Teese**

Question 10

Who is your favourite musician?

Is it them?
Is it their journey?
Is it their message?
Is it their story?
Is it their sound?
Is it a combination of all that they are?

Is it your memories?
Is it your emotion?
Is it your pleasure?
Is it your joy?
Is it your pain?
Is it combination of all that you are?

It is the entertainment?
Is it the triggers?
Is it the escape?
Is it the timing?

GET TO KNOW YOU

Is it the beat?
Is it about you or is it about them?

What do you love about your favourite musician?
What resonates with you?
What connects you to them?
What ties you forever to their music, to their story,
to their sound, to them?

Question 11
What is your favourite car?

If you love cars you will find this an easy question to answer. However, if cars are just a convenience to you, a practicality, a necessity, a way to get from A to B you may struggle. Even if this is the case for the moment just let your imagination soar.

What would be your dream car?
What colour?
What make?
What model?

Let your resistance drop and allow yourself to go wherever your heart and energy takes you. Now that you have allowed yourself to do that, I would encourage you, within the next week, to go to the showroom and sit in your dream car. See it, feel it, smell it, connect to it.

Call it to you!

GET TO KNOW YOU

How do you feel?
What emotions does just sitting in your dream car bring up for you?
What blocks or beliefs does sitting in this car reveal to you?
What stirs within you?

Allow yourself to feel!
Allow yourself to dream!
Allow yourself to feel worthy!
Allow the car to speak to you, to touch you.

Question 12

Where is your favourite holiday destination?

You may have visited and holidayed at this destination or you may have heard about it from others, seen it on a travel show or maybe dreamed about it. It doesn't matter.

What do you love about it or think you may love about it?
What are your favourite memories or why do you think you dream about it?
Is it the place or maybe the people you experienced it with that stands out most for you?
What feelings or emotions does, or would holidaying in that place trigger in you?

Do you long for adventure or relaxation, connection or freedom, the experience or the memories, the people or the places, the accommodation or the sights, the food or the vistas, the familiarity or the unusual, the comfort or the challenge?

GET TO KNOW YOU

Would it be an opportunity to 'be' you, or to discover you?

What is it about this destination, this experience, this holiday that you love or just know you would love?

Relive the memories or explore the dream.

Question 13

What is your favourite meal?

This is one of the questions my son asked me all those years ago and one that struck me really hard.

I had no idea. I couldn't answer him.

I couldn't believe I didn't even know what my favourite meal was!!!

And the look on my son's face touched something within me that told me this was important, that I needed to take this seriously.

How could a grown woman not even know what her favourite meal was!

Well I didn't; I had no idea, but as I committed to this journey and progressed through these questions, deepening my connection to self and improving my understanding of me, I slowly remembered.

Any meal that I don't have to cook myself is up there but my favourite meal is a creamy chicken risotto with shaved parmesan, rocket and a warm sour dough accompanied by a cool, crisp but light Rosé.

My mouth waters as I think of it.

I enjoyed a fabulous one some years ago and the taste of it stills lingers for me. I wait now in anticipation for one that beats it.

Question 14
What is your all-time favourite food?

I was challenged by today's question.

It seemed so similar to the previous question so I doubted its validity, its purpose, and its power. I thought, *I don't think I will include this one as people may think it is a double up or just a mistake.*

"STOP," echoed in my head.

I stopped and listened, and here is what came through. All of these questions were guided so I knew listening to the guidance in regard to them was important.

Here is the message I received exactly as I received it:

> *You are two weeks into this process now so the timing of this message is perfect. You may be loving the process, you may be doubting it, or you may be taking it for granted due to its apparent simplicity. You are used to expecting change to occur as the result of hard work, of huge effort, of struggle, of big actions!*

This is not always the case and with today's question we would like to explain something to you that we feel will serve you well not only through the rest of this journey but in life.

The power of these questions lies in their simplicity and in their subtle, small, differences.

The power of each question lies in the individual's willingness to consider the question. The answer is often not as powerful as the process you use to get to the answer!

The power lies in each person's desire and commitment to go deeply within themselves and find the answer, their answer.

The connection you seek lies in this process more than in each answer.

The power of subtlety is frequently lost on those of you going through this human experience as you are often keen to lump things together for the sake of ease, for the sake of time, and sometimes for the sake of hiding. You brush over the subtle differences because you don't see the point or subconsciously you don't want to delve that deeply into you!

You often like to generalise, to live on the surface, to grab the answer nearest and easiest. You humans love ticking boxes. A bit like in school … "I'm done Miss!" Often you think that is the goal, to be done, to complete something, when the true goal is to commit to the process.

You feel safe when you generalise, you feel you have room to move if someone disagrees with you, you feel free to change your mind, you feel safer, you feel less exposed but this just means you are being less authentic and less connected to you.

There is a difference between a meal and food, just like there is a difference between a piece of fabric and a piece of clothing, and as there is a difference between a flower and a tree. We (energy) see these differences as huge, yet you (humans) often want to put them all together and ignore the subtle variations for ease.

But ease of what?

As you walk through life we want you to start recognising, noticing and acting on the subtle differences; the slight difference in feeling when the direction you are heading, which once seemed perfect starts to feel a little off, a little uncomfortable; the small change of feelings in your gut; the subtle messages and thoughts we send you to help along the way. We want you to stop, reassess and listen to the subtle changes. If you do this, you could so often avoid major dramas, painful events, stress! These subtleties can help keep you on track, on your track, on your path.

Subtlety matters!

If you start seeing the differences in the questions we ask you this will start to draw your attention to the importance and the power of small things.

So often it is the small things that make the big things possible, that actually create the 'big' things in life. Small things matter, small changes in your feelings matter, small messages matter, small quiet thoughts matter.

Small is important.

Subtle differences are powerful!

Have you ever felt that slight change in the air and known a storm is brewing? The change is tiny, hard to describe, but you feel it, you sense it. The difference in the air is slight but the storm may be huge and if you 'listen' to the small change and get inside or put the car away or make whatever preparations you need to, the storm can pass with little impact on you. The warning was small, its impact huge.

Start paying more attention to the subtleties. Look inside of you for the true answer to the questions, to each question. Take a moment with each question, breathe and go within. Go below the surface.

Question 15
Who is your favourite actor?

A good actor, an actor who appeals to you, has the uncanny ability to transport you to another place and time, to draw you into a story, often triggering your own emotions or memories or even dreams.

Is it their skills or their personality or maybe even their quirkiness that touches you?
Maybe it is their ability to portray complex characters?
Possibly the genre of story they choose to help bring to life?
Is it the way they act or the way they live?
Is it this that touches you, that resonates with you, or is it something else?
What is it about your favourite actor that touches you, that appeals to you, or that stays with you?

"Acting is not about being famous, it's about exploring the human soul"

– Annette Benning

Question 16

What is your favourite sound?

How does this sound make you feel or what does the sound remind you of?
What memories or emotions does it stir within you?

Hands down, my favourite sound is rain on a tin roof or better still rain on a tin roof accompanied by the sounds of a storm.

As a child I found the sound comforting. To curl up in bed, snuggle under the blankets and listen to the rain, wind and even thunder outside, was bliss. I think it reminded me that we can be safe in seeming danger or even chaos. It started to teach me about my own ability to be calm inside as things raged around me.

The sound really brought me back to me! It still has a distinct effect on my emotions and sends goose bumps down my body.

How do you react to your favourite sound?
What does it trigger in you?

"It takes courage to grow up and become who you really are."

– E.E. Cummings

Question 17
What is your favourite emotion?

I have struggled with sharing this question. I experienced immense resistance to it and a reluctance to include it.

I decided not to include it, but it continued to take up an unreasonable amount of time in my thoughts indicating that I would benefit from looking at it further rather than just attempting to ignore it and move on!

I looked at the question and thought, w*ell everyone is going to answer love, or joy, or happiness, so what is the point in asking this one?* It didn't feel like a question that would help create any connections, light bulb moments or self-realisations.

I have asked, and questioned, and sat with it, and this is what came up.

It is important to consciously identify your 'favourite' emotion. How do you want to feel or wish you felt most of the time?

From what I have read it is fairly widely believed that there are only six or seven actual core emotions. Now you will find variances on this but it seems to be widely thought that all 'emotions' or 'feelings' fall under categories like:

Anger	Surprise
Fear	Disgust
Sadness	Hurt
Joy	

The categorisation of emotions is far from an exact science and you can find many different 'lists'. In fact I have included one such list over the page so you can see what I mean. This one actually has eight categories.

It outlines that while you may desire happiness, this might include the feelings of joy, optimism, calm, gratefulness etc. I interpret this to mean that there are varying degrees or manifestations of each core emotion.

Once you have answered honestly, "What is my favourite emotion/feeling?" ask yourself this, "What emotion do I sit in most often?"

Is this answer aligned, or congruent with your favourite emotion?

Now it starts to make sense, the power and the purpose of these questions begins to be revealed.

My favourite emotion for example is joy or happiness.

The emotion I sit in most often is fear!

Those two emotions are POLAR OPPOSITES!!

If I refer to the table on pages 42–43 I would find fear (or scared) under 'Insecure'.

Once I realised this, I received another message:

To get to joy, your desired emotion, you must let go of your obsession with fear (or insecurity or uncertainty), stop entertaining its presence, stop nurturing its energy, stop sitting in it, stop believing it. You will benefit from turning towards joy when the niggles of fear start within you.

With this realisation I accepted that I can choose my desired or favourite emotion rather than just wait for it to turn up! I can turn to it. I am not trapped in or by fear.

Then I looked at the list over the page and it dawned on me and this is powerful!

If joy seems a stretch when I am experiencing strong fear, I can reach for calm, or gratitude or hope. This will help 'bridge' the gap between fear, what I am feeling, and joy, what I wish to feel.

What do you wish to feel – and is that aligned or misaligned with what you feel most often?

FEELINGS WORD GUIDE

(http://jworldtimes.com/jwt2015/magazine-archives/jwtmag2018/july2018/english-for-css-pms-comprehension/)

Sad	Happy	Hurt	Helped
Depressed	Hopeful	Abused	Cherished
Lonely	Supported	Forgotten	Befriended
Disgusted	Charmed	Ignored	Appreciated
Angry	Grateful	Judged	Understood
Frustrated	Calm	Offended	Commended
Annoyed	Amused	Victimised	Empowered
Discouraged	Optimistic	Rejected	Accepted
Upset	Content	Cursed	Blessed
Despairing	Joyful	Destroyed	Healed
Uninterested	Enthusiastic	Hated	Loved
Disappointed	Thrilled	Despised	Esteemed
Hateful	Loving	Mistreated	Taken Care of
Bitter	Kind	Crushed	Reassured
Sorrowful	Celebratory	Injured	Made Whole
Mournful	Overjoyed	Tortured	Saved

Insecure	Confident	Tired	Energised
Weak	Strong	Indifferent	Determined
Hopeless	Brave	Bored	Inspired
Doubtful	Certain	Drained	Creative
Scared	Assured	Sick	Healthy
Anxious	Prepared	Exhausted	Renewed
Defeated	Successful	Dull	Vibrant
Worthless	Valuable	Weary	Alert
Guilty	Forgiven	Paralysed	Enlivened
Ugly	Beautiful	Powerless	Strengthened
Pressured	At Ease	Dejected	Motivated
Forced	Encouraged	Listless	Focussed
Stressed	Peaceful	Burned Out	Rejuvenated
Nervous	Relaxed	Fatigued	Invigorated
Worried	Secure	Blah	Animated
Embarrassed	Confident	Stale	Refreshed

"To become conscious and aware, we must become authentic and authenticity includes both positive and negative."

– Teal Swan

Question 18
Who is your favourite politician or political figure?

You may be shocked or a little confused to read this question. Politics is a conversation many of us avoid and respect of individual politicians is rare these days. This was another question I did not want to include and yet I was guided to so here it is.

It is my hope that this question may encourage you to look back and look around. You may be surrounded by politicians for whom you have little or no respect and the media is focussed on every negative angle, further diminishing any shred of respect we may have had. But broaden your view. Look beyond the current crop.

In the past we have had some politicians who showed great resilience, strength, honesty, passion, respect, flexibility, clarity, commitment, fairness, courage, knowledge, integrity and more.

We associate politicians with leadership and this question, if explored, will help you understand what traits you think make a good leader, what traits are you wishing to see in your leaders today. When we focus on these traits we may notice a new breed of politicians emerge.

And then, even more powerfully, you can identify the traits you believe you would need to be a positive leader because we are all leaders, whether that be leaders of ourselves or within our families or communities or workplace or broader, and if we step up we can change the world.

If you can't get past this question being about a politician and you can't come up with any maybe look at leaders.

Who is your favourite leader?

Question 19
Who was/is your favourite teacher?

As you recall teachers you have liked, teachers who have touched you, inspired you, and encouraged you, you will also undoubtedly remember some who have impacted you negatively, who let you down, who were less than inspiring.

When considering this question I encourage you to focus on those teachers who have impacted you in positive ways; those who opened your eyes to worlds you didn't know existed, who touched your soul in places you had never felt and who encouraged you to be you because being you was so awesome!

These may be classroom teachers, teachers of life, friends, work colleagues, family or partners. Teacher is not just a profession; teacher is a calling, and teaching is not restricted to classrooms.

Each and every one of you have opportunities to teach, and when you do, I encourage you to recall these positive teachers, your favourite teachers, and to think of their qualities, the impact they had on you, the difference they made. Each of you, at different times, in different ways, have opportunities to touch the lives of others.

Decide now what imprint you want to leave. You are, each of you, teachers!

Question 20
What is your favourite drink?

Getting to know you, strengthening your neural pathways so that thinking about you becomes easier, is aided by the simple things. The simple questions.

We are just exercising that 'muscle'.

As you reflect, think about and consider your favourite drink remember times you have enjoyed it, remember how it tastes, maybe go and have one now. Using all your senses helps build those links!

"You don't become what you want, you become what you believe."

– Oprah Winfrey

Question 21
What is your favourite animal?

Identify that one animal that stands out for you. It may change over time but the one that stands out for you right now will have a message for you.

Look up that animal and its symbolism. What does that animal represent? What are its traits? There will be a message in that for you ... maybe a trait you are denying could in fact be one of the keys to showing the world who you are. Something you deny in yourself perhaps?

When you read about it, something will stand out to you, something you can learn from your favourite animal.

There is a message for you that will help you move further along your path if you take the time to explore this.

What do you admire in this animal? It is probably a mirror for what is within you.

When I asked myself what my animal was, and allowed an answer to come, it was elephant. I searched elephant symbolism and energetic meanings ... parts of what I found really stood out for me and yes I got messages.

The strongest message I got from the elephant meaning and symbolism was that I would benefit from stepping into my wisdom; becoming the leader I have always desired to be. I am also stronger than I think! And I could step into the 'confidence' of the elephant.

You might be surprised by the messages your favourite animal reveals to you.

Question 22
What is your favourite flower?

Now you have identified your favourite flower, I am guided to ask you – do you use your flower?

Do you have them around you?
Do you treat yourself and buy them for yourself?
Do you look at them and smile?
Do you grow them?

Just looking at and enjoying your flower will help increase your vibration ... did you know that? How easy and what a beautiful way to raise your vibration, your energetic presence.

Walk into a florist, a market, or a nursery and pay attention to the vibrational feeling of the flowers.

Natural beauty is in the world for you to enjoy; do you enjoy these magical flowers as much as you could?

I also encourage you to look at the properties of your favourite flower's essence. You may be surprised at the alignment with your journey.

Do you realise most of your 'likes' aren't random? They often have a purpose to improve your life and experience!

These questions help you build your connection to self and rediscover who you are but they also provide you with vital information you can use everyday!

Question 23
What is your favourite tree?

Trees represent eternal life and can be a powerful tool to support your connection to source – God, spirit, angels, the universe, whatever you would like to call the divine.

Your 'totem' tree, usually identified as your favourite tree, is the tree that speaks to your heart, and can play a powerful role in grounding you. Touching the bark or trunk of your favourite tree can literally bring you home.

Meditating under your 'favourite' tree will help create a pure connection to the divine; the shadow of your favourite tree can actually shed light on your shadows. Under your favourite tree, in its shadow you can be you, the whole of you. The shadow of your tree is a powerful presence.

During meditation, you are often guided to go to a peaceful place, a place you like; may I suggest this place includes your favourite tree? Visualising or feeling this tree's presence in your meditationn will heighten and clarify your meditation.

Trees reach into the earth, they spread under your feet, they reach for the heavens, way way above our heads and they embrace the air.

Feel them!

Celebrate and acknowledge their presence.

Question 24
What is your favourite gift to receive?

This question can be particularly tricky for many people.

Are you accustomed to just settling for whatever you get or maybe nothing at all? Are you reluctant to identify what you love to receive as you feel it makes you less grateful for the other things you may be given? Do you not think, really believe, you are worthy of that which you would love to be given?

Do you know the problem may not be that you aren't given exactly what you desire; the problem could be that you can't accept what you truly desire, you don't feel worthy enough so you don't even explore or admit to yourself or anyone else what you truly would like to receive.

Identify what you want, what you would love, what you love to receive as a gift and then be open and willing to receive. So often you block it, you resist, you make excuses and you send it back!

DON'T!!

Be willing to accept.

Ask yourself, "Do I receive graciously and willingly. Am I truly open to receiving?"

Ask and really listen!

Are you ready to receive, ready to receive exactly what you want and love to receive?

But first, are you willing to ask, to be truthful about what you want and would love to receive?

Question 25

What is your favourite gift to give?

How does giving make you feel?
What feelings does it trigger for you?
Responsibility or freedom?
Resentment or love?
Lack or abundance?

The feelings behind your giving are just as important and in fact more important than what you give. It is the intention, not the gift, that touches people's hearts.

What gift do you most like to give?
Why?
Why do you think you particularly like giving this gift?

Gift giving is fairly simple. Give freely from your heart. That is the only rule that matters when giving.

"Don't trade your authenticity for approval."

– Anonymous

Question 26
What was your favourite birthday/birthday celebration?

Take a trip down memory lane.

Why was this particular birthday or birthday celebration so special?

Was it the people or the gifts, the celebration or the emotion, the accolades or the thoughts?

What stands out for you?

Celebrating another year of life is powerful and it should be done in a way that matters to you and touches your soul.

How do you most love to celebrate your special day?

If you avoid celebrations, especially those focused on you, why?

Ask yourself why?

What are you avoiding?

This can be particularly revealing. Many people avoid

personal celebrations to avoid being disappointed; perhaps this is you; perhaps you have a different reason.

Exploring your emotions and reactions around celebrating your own special day can be quite revealing.

Question 27
What is your favourite thing to cook?

What do you love about cooking this food or meal?
Is it the end result?
Do you enjoy sharing the meal?
Or maybe it is the smells and tastes?
Is it perhaps the memories it evokes?
Possibly a sense of accomplishment?

It may not be about the end result; it might be about the process.

Why do you love cooking this particular dish?

It isn't always about cooking the perfect meal or baking the best cake, it is about how you feel doing it.

"Cooking is all about people. Food is maybe the only universal thing that really has the power to bring everyone together. No matter what culture, everywhere around the world, people get together to eat."

– Guy Fieri

Question 28
Who is your favourite author?

I can hear some of the doubts and questions from here and yes I agree, some of these questions seem random and almost pointless at first.

"I have told you my favourite book; why does my favourite author matter?"

The resistance to delving deep into you and travelling along that less than familiar neural pathway can be very strong.

For some of these questions, their point can be found in the answer. The process of answering them honestly reveals parts of you that you have long ignored or forgotten. For others the point of the question is the process of searching for the answer. Remember, we are exercising a muscle and that can be aided by seemingly small, almost insignificant movements.

This is part of the 'training': the training you to think about you, the building of your neural pathway to self, the gathering and acknowledgement of knowledge about you. We are creating and nurturing a new habit. The habit of thinking about yourself, perhaps even thinking about you first!

Your favourite author may trigger something deep within you. Their words, journey or stories may touch you deeply.

Just as valuably though, they may just entertain you. Their writing may help you switch off for a little while, leave your cares behind and wrap yourself up in their stories and this can be just as valuable as anything they can teach you or reveal to you about yourself.

Entertainment has value; the ability to help you switch off and dream has immense value!

They may teach you, touch your heart, comfort you, remind you, calm you or entertain you.

Question 29
What is your favourite exercise?

Movement connects you to your physical body, the very vehicle that is allowing your soul to have this physical, human experience.

Movement, however subtle, honours your body and the connection you have to it.

Exercise doesn't need to be training for a marathon or swimming for an hour or smashing it out at a gym.

Walking, stretching, dancing, playing backyard cricket, throwing a ball for your dog, even pushing your child on a swing can all be ways of introducing exercise into your day.

Our bodies are designed to move and when we move we improve our physical state and the connection we have with our incredible bodies.

Knowing the type of exercise or movement that you like is important because you can start there and it won't feel like exercise; it will feel like fun; it will feel like you are just honouring you!

Building movement into your day in a way you enjoy is powerful!

There are physical, mental, emotional and spiritual benefits in movement. It is about so much more than getting physically fit even though that is fabulous.

Build exercise into your day, everyday, in fun ways and experience the difference on all levels.

Question 30

What is your favourite pen to write with?

"Who cares?" I hear you say. "A pen is a pen!"

Your answer may not be very telling but whether you use that pen is.

Many of us have pens in our bags, our cars, or at our desk, maybe even beside our bed. Wherever we write we tend to have pens.

Take a look right now.

What sort of pens are they?
What pens are you actually using?
What pens are you using to write your cheques, record your messages, pen your cards or sign your name?
Do you honour yourself enough to ensure you can always use your favourite pen?
Are you showing the universe your thoughts are worth that?
Are you showing the universe your money is worth that?
Are you showing the universe that your messages are worth that?

Are you showing the universe that your connection with loved ones is worth that?
Are you showing the universe that YOU are worth that?

A pen is a simple thing but simple things are often symbolic.

Honour yourself and your written word enough to whenever possible use your favourite pen. If you don't why are you settling? Then ask yourself what else are you settling on? What other areas of your life are you compromising on and selling yourself short?

Question 31
What is your favourite metal?

Metals carry their own symbolic meanings and energetic properties and we can be drawn to particular metals due to their unique properties. Some people even believe that metals hold magical properties.

It can be really interesting to look into the meanings and properties of your favourite metal and see if there is a deeper message for you.

You can use metals, much like crystals, to aid your spiritual growth and path.

For example, copper can be used to help alleviate negative energy; platinum can aid wisdom; zinc can assist in times of transition; aluminium can be useful for energetic protection.

If you want to look further into metals, especially your favourite metal, and how you could work with it there are many websites that explore this in depth.

A google search for 'energetic properties of metals' will find many websites exploring this topic.

"Success is liking yourself, liking what you do, and liking how you do it."

– **Maya Angelou**

Question 32
What is your favourite crystal?

Every natural substance, including crystals, have a unique vibration that creates their own energy.

What you are drawn to could be the energy that naturally radiates from the crystal, the same energy that gives it unique properties. This energy may align with yours or maybe even help raise your own energy improving your energetic state. The energy of the crystal may even have a healing ability that you would currently benefit from.

The trick is knowing what they truly are and trusting that they aren't just random.

Through this process you are discovering exactly what your preferences are by asking yourself questions you may have never asked.

Wherever possible surround yourself with that which you like, that which you love, that which makes you smile and that which speaks to you!

"There will always be someone who can't see your worth."

"Don't let it be you."

– Mel Robbins

Question 33
What is your favourite activity/hobby?

Putting time aside to indulge in your hobbies, to even explore new hobbies, is a valuable component of self-care.

While engaged in hobbies and activities you enjoy, with no intentions or desired outcome other than to relax and have fun, you naturally and effortlessly connect with your inner self.

Taking time to enjoy your hobbies is not just a powerful way to honour yourself, it is fun and you deserve to have fun. You can never have too much fun in your life!

Do what you love and love what you do.

Make time for all the things you love, your life will thank you for it.

"Aren't you a little sick and tired, by now, of holding back your brilliance, in order not to offend or unsettle people?"

– **Katrina Ruth**

Question 34
What is your favourite sport?

You may watch it, you may play it, or you may have played it in the past.

It doesn't matter.

Sport can be a fun way to get physically active, connect with others and learn new skills, even to challenge and push yourself.

Watching a sport you love can be a great stress reliever, an escape or just a way to have fun. Watching and following sport can help you connect with other people through your mutual interest.

Fun is undervalued and often ignored as reason enough to do something.

Fun leads to increased energy, decreased stress, greater productivity and connection, improved positivity and so much more.

Not a sport lover?

GET TO KNOW YOU

This is going to sound a little weird but instead ask this.

Which sport do you most dislike?

Remember the aim of this whole process is to connect to you.

Sure it is great to do that in positive ways but even exploring what we don't like builds that link to self!

Question 35
What is your favourite subject?

This subject doesn't need to be linked to your work and in fact it often isn't. Exploring topics outside of your profession, just for the fun of it, helps expand your mind and energy.

It doesn't matter what the subject is; exploring topics that interest and excite you adds another dimension to who you are.

What is a subject you love to learn about and talk about?
What subject do you feel you can lose yourself in?
Do you explore it?
Do you talk about it?

Maybe you should, you may be surprised where it leads you and what connections it helps you make.

And again have fun with it … having fun has been a bit of a theme with the last few questions, don't forget to have fun with this whole process.

"Be yourself, everyone else is taken."

– Oscar Wilde

Question 36

What is your favourite herb?

When I was first asked this question I was guided to look up the health benefits of coriander, my favourite herb.

As I was reading through the many health benefits of this beautiful herb I was struck by the fact it helps with anaemia or low iron.

I have been prone to anaemia on and off over the years and had been feeling really tired. Not just a little weary every now and then, bone tired most days and sometimes almost as soon as I wake up.

I didn't click that it could be low iron again.

Thank you coriander for this awareness!

Look up the amazing health benefits of your favourite herb. There might be a message in it for you too!

"Just be yourself, there is no one better."

— **Taylor Swift**

Question 37

What is your favourite shell?

Did you know that throughout time shells have been used in magic and primarily in magic that is used to draw things you desire to you?

This means they can be used in manifestation, to support and strengthen the law of attraction!

When you have your favourite shells around your home, or include them in any of your rituals you can magnify your manifesting ability.

Shells are especially powerful in areas of love and prosperity! It is believed by some, that a small shell kept in your wallet is thought to attract money, and it can help to keep the money flowing in.

Shells also represent protection and have strong protection energy.

Combining shells, especially your favourite shells, with your crystals can be very powerful. And they are beautiful so it is a win-win!

Do you have your favourite shells in your home?

"To be beautiful means to be yourself. You don't need to be accepted by others. You need to accept yourself."

— **Thich Nhat Hanh**

Question 38
What makes you smile?

A smile, a real smile, is powerful. Smiling can positively affect how you feel and even how those around you feel, interact with and perceive you. A simple smile can have a major impact on your experiences.

Smiling can lift your vibration, change your focus and even positively influence those around you. Hopefully you smile often, but do you know what actually makes you smile?

When I first contemplated this question, I was going to answer, "my children". Especially when they do certain things. Like if I am in another room yet I can over hear them chatting, laughing and cheering each other on; that always makes me smile.

But then I stopped. Some time ago I realised that I needed to stop relying on my children for my happiness and my purpose. I could talk about my thoughts on this at length but I realised it was unfair on them and on me to rely on them for this basic desire – happiness. They didn't need that pressure! And I needed to take responsibility for my happiness in a way I could control, not give that control to someone else. My children are my priority, but if I put them too firmly at the centre of who I am, they have no room to grow, it is stifling!!

I wondered, could this question about smiling be similar?

Smiling is so powerful and a really valuable part of my day. What if the kids are fighting and being right little sh**ts as they can be, does that mean I won't authentically smile that day? Does that mean they have 'taken away' my reason to smile? Again too much pressure!

I was guided to think deeper. What really made me smile from the inside and wasn't reliant on other people?

In the morning, when the house is quiet and I make that first cup of tea and I hold that cup in my hands and breathe … I smile. I smile from within me.

Standing watching a beautiful sunset or sunrise, allowing its absolute magnificence to touch me, I smile. I truly smile.

Being aware of small things that make you smile, a memory, a song, a certain sound, a photo, and then consciously drawing on those memories, activities or experiences can help put an authentic smile on your face just when you need to.

Question 39
What makes you laugh?

It seems even science now supports the fact that laughter has health benefits, both physical and mental. The benefits of laughter are thought to include:

Lowering blood pressure.
Reducing stress hormone levels.
Releasing the body's feel-good hormones.
Helping reduce the risk of cancer.
Increasing creativity.
Boosting the immune system.
Improving memory.
Improving mood.
Exercising your abdominal and facial muscles.

As well as these benefits, it just feels good. Who doesn't love a good deep laugh?

We have a video of my daughter on a slingshot ride; just the thought of it makes me laugh, watching it sees me in fits of laughter with tears streaming down my face every time. As I sit here typing this I can't help but laugh about it and I haven't even watched it for over 2 years!!

When I know I could use a laugh, I can think of that or I sit down and watch *The Big Bang Theory*; it always makes me laugh!

Knowing what makes you laugh means you can use it to your advantage and when you need to you can have a really good laugh. It feels good to laugh, it can break a bad mood or halt a negative spiral and I would personally embrace any of benefits listed previously.

Make sure you let yourself laugh, the more often and the deeper the better.

Question 40
What makes you cry?

As you progress through these questions, are they becoming easier to answer? Are you curious to know what your answer is rather than questioning why the question has been asked?

Are you enjoying the process of giving yourself permission to think about you? Are you loving finding out about you and asking yourself questions you may never have asked before?

The more you surrender to the process the more powerful it will be.

A little like crying really. When you surrender to the need to cry, to the urge to cry and allow tears to flow they help facilitate a powerful release.

Do you allow yourself to cry?
Do you cry around others?
Do you judge your own tears or label them as a sign of weakness?
Do you judge the tears of others?

Do you shy away from the vulnerability tears can make you feel?

Crying not only has physical benefits for the eyes and even the body it has emotional benefits. Crying has actually been found to improve your mood, it can dull pain, it may assist in restoring emotional balance, it is a necessary stage of grief and crying has a soothing effect.

Crying is not a sign of weakness it can in fact be a sign of strength and it can also be a sign of authenticity. *Not* crying doesn't make you strong!

Question 41
What makes you scared?

Being scared can hold you back.
Being scared can be a habit.
Being scared is often based on the past.

Do you regularly feel scared, or is fear easily triggered within you? Ask yourself:

Am I in danger?
Is this fear helpful?
Is this fear current?
Is this fear justified?
Is this fear real?
Is this fear mine?

Based on your answers you may find you are responding from an old pattern, habit or memory and it might be time to acknowledge, challenge and release the fear.

Being 'fearless' is a big call and I don't aim for it.

Fear can be beneficial; sometimes it is a great warning and we may need it to survive, but not very often. For the most part we have become too comfortable (even though it feels uncomfortable) sitting in and listening to our fear. Many people focus far too much time and energy on their fear.

Personally, I have accepted I will always feel fear but I have also decided to accept that I don't have to listen to it, I don't have to be guided by it or limited by it. In fact I can act in spite of it.

Fear has taken away enough opportunities from me and it is time to take that power back.

What about you?
Could you benefit from listening less to your fears?

Question 42
What makes you jump for joy?

Many people dampen or play down and contain their expressions of joy, and therefore their experience of joy. They don't let those moments of pure joy descend on them.

Do you allow yourself this level of emotion?
Do you allow yourself to experience and demonstrate joy?
Have you ever experienced this?
Do you stifle your joy?
If so why do you do this?

Maybe you have been taught to. Perhaps you don't want to boast or be seen as egotistical. Do you fear what others may think? Possibly you don't want to offend others who may not feel as joyful as you do at the time.

We are all born with a natural compulsion to 'jump for joy'; you can observe it in children. They do it naturally and unapologetically.

Maybe it is time you rediscovered that feeling.

If you can't remember the last time you literally 'jumped for joy' think about what would possibly make you feel like 'jumping for joy'. You may need to go way back, back to a time in your childhood even. If you can't recall a time imagine what it would feel like to jump for joy and what might trigger that within you.

Remember joy happens in moments, joy comes out of nowhere, joy can be fleeting but so powerful. It is different to the slow burn of happiness.

Does this question make you retreat and hide, or does it stir up feelings or memories of joy or perhaps the desire to feel that level of joy?

I had to dig, really dig deeply to find my answer.

Congratulations

You have completed six weeks of the 'Get to Know You' program.

I hope you are enjoying the time you are investing connecting with and thinking about you.

You have probably explored something already that you never thought of and with each question, you 'get to know you' a little bit more, a little bit deeper.

You may have noticed in the last few days there has been a gentle shift in the questions; they have moved towards feelings and emotions rather than just identifying 'things' you like. This shift continues as we move through the questions. Don't worry, it is a gradual change, but you may notice they become deeper, a bit more intimate or personal, some more thought-provoking and with that they may also trigger you. Please know you can handle that!

Be gentle on yourself and remain committed to being true to you. There are no right or wrong answers; just your answers. Some may be very obvious, and others may surprise you.

The real key as you move forward in this process is allowing your answers to come to you, to really listen to your own voice within. You hold all your answers; no one knows your answers as well as you and sometimes we forget that.

Over the next sixty days I suspect some of your answers may surprise you; the questions might too. Trust, sit with them, and don't dismiss them.

I recommend before you ask yourself each question you place your feet firmly on the ground or floor, take three deep and deliberate breaths and feel your heart or centre. Bring your awareness to that point within you, then ask the question and allow the answer to come from within you.

This is about discovering your deep truths, even if they are different from what you expected. Even when they are unexpected, there will be a level of knowing. You may be shocked or surprised by your answer, but you will just know it is true.

If you struggle with this approach, the following quick exercise might help you receive your answers rather than think them; it helps you see and 'feel' the difference between allowing and thinking an answer.

Let's imagine I ask you, "On a level of one to ten, one being not at all and ten being the highest possible, how happy are you right now?" What would you say?

A number will just come to mind. You don't have to think about it; the number just 'drops' into you, you just know it even though you didn't know you knew it. You don't know how you know, you just know.

On the other hand if I said, "So tell me what you did last Thursday", you would think about it and you would come up with an answer based on your memory and your conscious thoughts about what you did that day. You would recall the answer, much like you have with some of the preceding questions.

Many of the questions coming up require you to respond in the first way I described: you need to allow the answer to come to you, to come into your awareness; you don't think it or create it, you receive it.

See if you can feel and identify the difference in the way you access your answers. Approach the following questions with interest and openness.

Most importantly have fun!

Question 43
What makes you retreat?

I often retreat from my own truth or from change. It wasn't easy to admit to either of these responses but when I did, I realised that awareness was the first step to changing the habit. I do find it funny that I retreat from truth and change because truth, especially my own self-truth, and change, especially growth (which requires a willingness to change), are two of my strongest desires.

Yes, we sometimes retreat from the very things we desire!

There are occasions when we retreat for positive reasons or at least there are times when we could benefit from retreating. Sometimes we need to retreat to heal, to regroup, to reassess. This can definitely be a positive side of retreating as long as you know when to remerge.

Ask yourself, "Am I retreating to avoid something or am I retreating to gather the strength and clarity I need to face something?"

"You deserve to be happy, you deserve to be joyful, you deserve to be celebrated. But in order to do that you must first fall madly in love with yourself."

— **Lisa Nichols**

Question 44
What makes you hide?

I was confused by today's question. I thought it was the same or at least very similar to 'what makes you retreat?'

Apparently not.

Retreating and hiding are two very different things.

To retreat, you must have first surged or at least stepped forward. You must have attempted to face, tackle or deal with something and then, for any number of reasons, you decide to retreat.

Retreating can, in fact, be a good option. It can save you. It can allow you to step back and reassess. Usually when you retreat, you have faced something and taken on new information. You sometimes retreat to just regroup, gather strength or reassess and plan. This can be vital and even a very wise decision. Retreating can be self-protection or preservation.

Hiding, on the other hand, is different. You choose to not face something; you decide to ignore it instead. Hiding is rarely about truth, or strength, or even authenticity, and retreating CAN be all of these things, depending on what you do once you regroup of course; you can retreat and then choose to hide which then isn't constructive. Hiding is usually about fear and is often based on out-dated beliefs and limits.

Hiding is denial or attempted denial. Hiding is due to a lack of self-belief. Hiding is allowing fear to guide and direct you.

Can you see that hiding and retreating are actually different things? Both can be destructive, or at the very least unproductive, but retreating can also be a necessary, healing and a powerful step to move forward.

Hiding is rarely, if ever, positive.

So what do you hide from?

Question 45
What makes you dance?

I struggle with this one, because I feel so self-conscious when I dance; I always have. When I was a young teenager, I overheard a group of friends, my best friends, talking about how bad I was at dancing.

I was devastated.

I wasn't angry, as I knew what they said was true, but I was hurt by what I heard. I was sad because I knew it to be true and I so wanted it not to be. I wanted to be one of those who looked comfortable and 'cool' on the dance floor. Sadly I never have been, but that doesn't mean I don't love to dance … at times. I do have to really let go of caring what anyone else may think and that does take a lot of work (or perhaps even a few wines!).

When you truly allow yourself to dance, when you surrender to the music, the rhythm, the movement and the joy, you are able to release all judgement and expectations. You allow yourself to 'be'. To be present in the moment, to be present in your body, to be present in your energy. It is a fabulous way to feel present, present in the moment, in the now!

A unique connection can occur in that moment. A connection between the physical and the spiritual or energetic.

And it can be a whole lot of fun!

Surrender to the dance!

Question 46
What are you hiding?

This question made me nervous to share. It seemed so very personal and I feared people might shut down when faced with it. I thought at the very least people would avoid it. After all, they were hiding this 'thing' for a reason, and was a simple question going to have any bearing on them finally sharing it or even admitting to hiding it in the first place?

I shared it anyway and the first time I ran the 'Get to Know You' program, I forced myself to not just answer it but to share my answer.

I am going to share that answer here in the hope that it might encourage you to dig deeply within yourself and bring out what you too have been hiding. Why is this important? Shame lives in the darkness of denial and by ignoring and hiding something it doesn't deem it powerless; in fact it often has more power over us from those depths. So often bringing it into the light is when we can start to heal from it and take back our own power.

What am I hiding?

I have hidden sexual abuse as a child for a long time. It is seemingly more and more important to acknowledge that as a part of my experience. It is interesting that as I did that, as I acknowledged this experience, it become less and less powerful and significant. The darkness and denial, the hiding, had helped keep it alive!

And I hide, even from myself, the depth of my desire to share my thoughts and messages, my wisdom. I have for so long wanted to be an inspirational speaker and author and while I talk about it to some, I have hidden, from myself even, the strength of those desires for fear that people will think I am not good enough, not smart enough, not capable enough, or not knowledgeable enough. I also hide the strength of my desire and dream for fear people will laugh at me or ridicule me behind my back, especially if I fail.

In doing this I have unintentionally hidden me, the real me, the whole me, and it is time to stop doing that!

When you stand true in who you really are, all of you, the past loses power and when you authentically own your own unique desires and passions incredible opportunities can finally open up to you!

What are you hiding and what is it costing you?

Question 47
What makes you reflect?

We can reflect on positive or negative experiences, on what was or what might have been, on ourselves and on others.

Reflection brings learning to life and all experiences are an opportunity to learn. Reflection is an opportunity for feedback, a time to consider your actions, a way of cementing learning and an incredible opportunity to identify areas of improvement.

Reflection is careful, gentle, hopefully unbiased thought given to a situation, person, behaviour, event or self. You can reflect 'in' action, when you are in a situation, or 'on' action, after a situation has occurred and you are able to step back. Either way careful reflection can help shape your future decisions, actions and path. It can also help you gain perspective and clarity about people, events and situations. Reflection aids clarity and clarity helps us move forward with more confidence building a feeling of fulfilment and personal purpose.

"Don't ever let a soul in the world tell you that you can't be exactly who you are."

– **Lady Gaga**
(Stefani Joanne Angelina Germanotta)

Question 48
What makes you feel confident?

This sounds so simple and yet many people find it challenging to answer. Confidence, especially in self, is a big hurdle for many people.

When I first considered this question I sat with it thinking, *what gives me confidence?* But the truth is that nothing can 'give' me confidence except maybe myself, so I didn't know how to answer it.

Then I realised that wasn't the question, and that is a really important thing about all of these questions. You need to read what they are actually asking, not what you think they are asking. I thought it said, 'What gives you confidence?' when what it actually says is, "What makes you feel confident?" These are two different things.

You have confidence within you; you came into this life with confidence, confidence in your ability to be yourself, to walk your path, learn your lessons, make an impact and feel fulfilled and be personally successful. In fact, you were full of confidence. You now just need to tap into that again. Feel it again. To acknowledge your inner confidence!

What helps you feel your innate confidence?
What people, or situations, or thoughts, or actions help your feelings of confidence?

Question 49
What makes you doubt yourself?

As talked about in the previous question we are born with innate confidence. Confidence in who we are and our ability to navigate our own journey. Along the way we inevitably face challenges and we begin to doubt our own knowing, our path, our ability, ourselves. Some of us listen to these doubts too often and we begin to be guided by our doubts, or the doubts of others, and not our knowing and truth.

Knowing what or who triggers these doubts can really help you confront them and move forward on your path in spite of them. It isn't unusual to feel doubt but you won't achieve all you are capable of if you listen to it! Awareness is key to getting past the doubt and to clear it or to act in spite of it.

Is it time to stop listening to and being guided by your doubt?

"Doubt kills more dreams that failure ever will."

– **Suzy Kassem**

Question 50
What gets you talking?

We talk for a wide variety of reasons:

To communicate with others.
To connect with others.
To seek information.
To share information.
To express ourselves – our thoughts, feelings, opinions or ideas.
To explore a topic or to ask a question.
To be heard.
To distract ourselves from situations or even feelings.
To fill an uncomfortable silence.

I am sure there are other reasons, but this shows how important talking can be. Many of us however are quiet or have at least quietened our voice for fear of being wrong or offending others or of being ridiculed or harshly judged. Often, we pick 'safe' times to talk, people to talk to and subjects to talk about. Sometimes we even deliberately choose and censor our own words.

What gets you talking?
Authentically talking, sharing freely?
What emotions, people, situations, topics or environments give you the confidence to not just talk but talk freely, authentically, and passionately?

Question 51
What is your favourite personal attribute?

Does this question immediately make you feel uncomfortable?
Do you struggle to answer it honestly?
Do you feel resistance to even asking the question let alone answering it?
Can you easily identify all the things you don't like about yourself but struggle with admitting or even knowing what you do like?

If this is you it is time to stop! Stop being so readily critical of yourself. Decide to stop. Step back and observe yourself – your physical self, your personality, your actions.

Look into your eyes, see your smile, notice your hair or your fingers or your legs or your bum or maybe your nails. What about your personality traits?

GET TO KNOW YOU

Are you: caring, determined, kind, calm, loving, strong, reliable, cheerful, courageous, hardworking? The list could go on.

Really look at yourself. Look physically but also look deeply at who you are. See the incredible being others can see.

Refuse to be critical and allow yourself to be loving and accepting.

Now what is your favourite personal attribute?

You may even have many! Be proud of them, you can't be proud of what you don't acknowledge.

Question 52
As a child what did you dream of being when you grew up?

I love the way children talk so freely about what they want to be, what they truly believe they will be, when they grow up.

They speak with the same conviction whether they want to be an astronaut or a cleaner. To them all that matters is that in that moment they see it as being something that they would have fun doing. They also allow it to change as their own likes, desires and focus changes. One day they talk passionately about being a vet and the next they speak just as passionately about working in a coffee shop.

They don't worry in that moment how it will happen they just allow their hearts to speak.

Have you ever asked a child why they want to do the thing they say they want to do when they grow up?

It is really interesting they so often answer with things like:

I want to help people.
I like keeping things clean.
I love animals.
I like talking to people.
People are happy when they get their coffee.

These answers seem general and a little simplistic, but they can reveal a lot about not just what someone likes to do but what they are good at. They are answers given from the heart.

Childhood dreams were dreamed without judgement and limits. You were just as likely to have wanted to be a garbage man as a scientist or a sailor as a doctor, or a cleaner as a super hero.

Your dreams were often based on what looked fun, what you liked doing or maybe on saving the world!

What did you want to be when you grew up and why?
Why did you think you would like it and would be good at it?
What does this reveal to you about you?

Can you learn anything from your answers?

Question 53
What do you feel is your weakness?

This was another of the questions I was reluctant to share when it was first given to me and I asked, "Should we really draw attention to someone's perceived weakness? Should we give our weaknesses even a moment of our time?"

Here is the answer I received:

Just like there is light and dark, happy and sad, full and empty, there are strengths and weaknesses. It is you who judges a weakness as a negative thing; we just see it as what is at the moment, another part of the amazing individual each of you are.

Being aware of your weakness does not give it strength; being aware and bringing it into the light means you can accept it as part of who you are, managing it as you walk your path or, if you choose, you can work on it.

Everyone has weaknesses; without them you can't have strengths. It is time to release the shame and denial humans often have around them.

So what is your weakness?

Maybe if you are lucky, you can identify more than one!

Question 54
What do you, or could you do, to overcome your weakness?

First ask yourself, "Do I wish to overcome this perceived weakness? Would I benefit from working on it?"

Without sensing a benefit to us, it just feels like hard work and something we will often give up on when it gets hard or challenging. We might place it on our pile of failures to reflect on or even obsess over when we feel down or 'less than', adding unhelpfully to those feelings.

If you feel there is a benefit to working on or overcoming your weakness, ask yourself, "Does it really matter?" "How does this affect me?" "Do my strengths more than compensate for this?"

You may get to a place where you can actually accept and even love your weakness.

One of my weaknesses is self-doubt; this weakness doesn't serve me in any way. I use my awareness to overcome it and at times refuse to listen to it or be guided by it but it is a constant process for me.

Another 'weakness' I have is I often care too much about others, sometimes more than they seem to care. I have addressed this and this 'weakness' is one I am happy to accept and am prepared to live with. My intuition is really helping me manage this!

Are you prepared to embrace and live with your 'weakness' or do you know it holds you back?

If it holds you back ask yourself, "What can I do to overcome this?" The answer is within you; you have probably just ignored it for a long time.

Question 55
What inspires, drives or motivates you?

Knowing what inspires, drives or motivates you can be one of your most powerful tools.

When you know what motivates you to grow and develop and do the work that needs to be done you can use that to your advantage.

Everyone has challenging days, days that lead you to doubt your path or even yourself, times when you seriously consider throwing in the towel, giving up.

When you know what inspires you, drives you or motivates you, you can turn to that when you need it most.

The best motivation comes from within. Knowing what triggers that sense of motivation from within you is more valuable than gold!

"There is nothing more rare, nor more beautiful, than a woman being unapologetically herself; comfortable in her perfect imperfection. To me, that is the true essence of beauty."

– Dr Steve Maraboli

Question 56
What holds you back?

This question is usually followed by a wide range of answers:

Lack of confidence or clarity.
Not knowing enough.
Risk of failure.
Judgement of others.
Self-doubt.
Overthinking.
Illness.

The list goes on but can you feel the common denominator here?
Fear.
Each one of these reasons is based on fear: fear of not being good enough, fear of failing, fear of judgment.

Ask yourself, "Is this fear founded on truth?" "Is this fear worth sacrificing my dreams for?" "Could I focus on faith and not fear?" "Do I really want fear dictating and guiding my future?"

For some of us, fear will always be present. Listening to your fear may have become an unhelpful habit, one that you can change.

Is this fear worth sacrificing your potential future?

Regardless of what is holding you back ask yourself, "Is it really worth it? Is it really worth listening to this fear?"

Question 57
Who supports you?

'Support' means different things to different people.

It can be someone who listens quietly.
Someone who gives feedback.
Someone who empathises.
Someone who pushes you.

It can be one person, or a small group of people, or for others it may be a large group of people. Some people need small support systems while others thrive on large groups of support people.

Receiving support is a basic human need and in no way indicates weakness. Quite often, reaching out for the support you need requires strength.

Studies have shown that social support can in fact reduce depression and anxiety. To benefit from that though you must know who not just supports you but who you feel supported by. Knowing who you can call on, who you can rely on for support is extremely valuable as you navigate this journey called life.

Don't ever be afraid to ask for help.

Reach out, most people love providing welcomed support to others.

Question 58
Who helps bring out the best in you?

It would be great if we all realised that it is up to us to bring out the best in ourselves, but as we learned yesterday, we sometimes need support.

This is especially powerful when you are down or life is feeling particularly tough or unfair. It is incredibly powerful to know who you can turn to, not to fix everything, but the person you can turn to who will help you see your strengths and successes. Someone who helps you dig deeply within to see your own potential and positive attributes.

Some people naturally help us see ourselves as more capable, and more amazing than we were seeing ourselves. These people will often be the ones that push us when we need it.

And once they help bring the 'best you' to the light, once they help you recognise all you are and all you can be you can stand up and work to bring the best out of yourself.

"To be yourself in a world that is constantly trying to make you something else is the greatest accomplishment."

– Ralph Waldo Emerson

Question 59
Who challenges you?

Do you see challenge as a positive or negative thing? Interestingly most people interpret this question as 'who challenges me negatively?'

We often see someone who challenges us as someone who questions what we do or who we say we are. It can feel like they are constantly trying to be 'better' than us or undermine us.

If this is the person who comes to mind, I would be asking, "What is the value of them in my life?" or, "Why do I keep inviting them into my life?" or, "Why do I listen to them?"

These answers may be revealing and even empowering; they may tell you a lot about yourself.

Challenge isn't always a negative thing though.

This person may challenge you to be the best you can be or to see your amazing potential and attributes. They might challenge you to grow and evolve.

Challenge can be confronting but it can also be positive.

"Never be bullied into silence. Never allow yourself to be made a victim. Accept no one's definition of your life; define yourself."

– Harvey Fierstein

Question 60
Who teaches you the most?

No teacher can teach without willing students.

Be a willing student and the teacher will appear. Not always in the way or as the person you expected. If you want to learn, be open to the teacher who appears; so often they are the right teacher for you at that time.

While life is a great teacher, and I think I would say my greatest teacher, it doesn't do it alone. The universe engages the services of people, places, experiences, emotions and even things to teach you what you need to learn, what you will benefit from learning.

Teachers can and do take many forms.

Are you ready to learn?

"When you are content to be simply yourself and don't compare or compete, everyone will respect you."

— **Lao Tzu**

Question 61
How do you best learn?

Recognising how we learn can help us embrace learning experiences.

Knowing there are many ways to learn may open us up to learning more quickly and possibly less painfully. It also helps us realise that others may learn differently from us. There is no perfect way to learn, however, there are easier ways for each individual to learn.

We can learn through instruction or being told what to do. We also learn through:

Mistakes.
Observation.
Reading.
Repetition.
Doing.
Hearing.
Discussion.
Reflection.
Trial and error.

GET TO KNOW YOU

How do you learn?
Is the way you are trying to learn serving you well?
Are you perhaps resisting the way or means that teaches you best?

Question 62
What do you 'beat' yourself up about?

How do you feel when you make a mistake, when things don't go well?

I admit I haven't always handled it well!
I have beaten myself up.
I have felt inadequate.
I have questioned my abilities.
Quite often I hide.

If I thought I said the wrong thing, I would then shut down; if I felt I did the wrong thing, the guilt would plague me even after I had apologised.

Putting myself out there online magnified this.

A few times I posted something online and almost immediately someone pointed out something like a spelling mistake. I would feel sick to my stomach, I would change it instantly, withdraw, and berate myself. I would allow feelings of inadequacy to grow. One day someone pointed out a spelling mistake on a meme I had created and shared. I immediately removed it and I didn't share another meme for months.

What power I gave my mistakes!

Then I saw something. An influencer with millions of followers posted a meme and in it he spelt health 'healt'. It was an obvious mistake in bold writing going out to millions of people.

That post got over 27,000 likes and was shared over 6,000 times. Yes some people pointed out his mistake, some kindly and some very rudely, but here is what struck me:

He didn't change it, he didn't take it down.

In fact the post is still there over two years later.

He posted more that day, he posted the next day, he kept sharing, and he possibly kept making mistakes, and he has kept growing. His reach has grown, his following has grown. His mistake didn't define him, he didn't let it. He didn't beat himself up about it!

I am sharing this with you not to highlight someone else's mistake but to highlight the fact he obviously doesn't beat himself up about his mistakes. He doesn't define himself by them. He accepts them as part of his journey!

If you don't allow yourself to make mistakes you won't do anything!!! And you certainly won't grow!

Whatever it is that you beat yourself up about I am sure there is a different way of looking at it if you allow yourself to!

Question 63
What was a major turning point in your life?

Turning points.

We all experience events in our lives when things change; they are necessary and inevitable. We change, and from that moment on we will never be exactly the same again.

Those turning points could be the beginning or end of a relationship, or:

Births	Moving
Deaths	Spiritual realisations
Marriages	Bankruptcy
Trauma	Retirement
Redundancy	Graduation

This list is only a start; everyone experiences different turning points. They can seem positive or negative. Both are a part of life but they change our thoughts, our beliefs, our direction and maybe even who we are.

These turning points can create moments of clarity, moments when we see things differently. Often we can look back on these points in life and gain an understanding about where we are now, who we are and maybe even our behaviours and beliefs.

You may have had control over some turning points, and you may have made decisions that led to them; others you might have had no control over; some were perhaps even controlled by other people and their actions.

Now though, as you stand and look at these turning points, realise that any moment could be a turning point in your life. Any moment you can choose to act differently than you are now, to look at things differently, to make different choices than you currently are.

Some turning points happen to us, others you control and you can choose to turn in a different direction any time.

Is what you are doing, the actions you are taking, what you are choosing to believe serving you right now?

If it isn't working for you, you can choose to make this moment a turning point in your life!

Question 64

Do you like tea or coffee, mugs or cups, tea bags or teapot, instant or ground?

Today's question is a fun and light one, a great question after yesterday.

Sharing and enjoying warm beverages is a ritual that has been observed, shared and passed down throughout the ages and across borders of countries and even across different beliefs.

Many of the world's problems or at least the challenges of a family have been discussed and even solved over a pot of tea or a cup of coffee.

Whether you drink it on the run, share it in a leisurely way with friends and family, sit and enjoy it at home or at your favourite coffee shop, I encourage you to take a moment and think about what you love about your favourite warm beverage.

Is it the taste, the ritual, the feelings, the memories or something else?

Take time to enjoy your favourite beverage in the way you enjoy it most.

"Always be a first-rate version of your yourself instead of a second-rate version of someone else."

– Judy Garland (Frances Ethel Gumm)

Question 65
Where is your dream location to live?

We all have them, locations we dream of living. It may be just down the road from where you currently live or across town. It might be in a different city or even a different country.

What is stopping you moving there?
Do you plan to move there one day?
What do you think would be different in your life if you lived in this location?
How do you think you would feel in this location?
How can you bring those feelings into your current home or location?

Have fun with this question. Don't limit yourself or your dream. Visualise it, write about it, think about it, but most importantly have fun with it.

"About all you can do in life is be who you are. Some people will love you for you. Most will love you for what you can do for them, and some won't like you at all."

– Rita Mae Brown

Question 66
What is your biggest success to date?

Sometimes we struggle to 'feel' successful in the now as we are striving for something other than what we are currently experiencing or something we are yet to experience. We are so often seeking some other level of success than that which we have already experienced or feel we have experienced. In that pursuit we can easily forget our past successes, forget we have been successful in the past and more importantly forget the feeling of actually being successful.

We constantly change our own goalposts and while this can be positive, pushing us to grow and reach our potential, it can also be detrimental if we never stop and enjoy and acknowledge our successes along the way, if we don't allow ourselves to feel successful!

GET TO KNOW YOU

So many people are constantly 'striving' (which is an external, lacking[1] and future based action and energy) for success.

They speak and act like success is something they are reaching for and have not yet attained: "When I am successful I will …" or "I want to be successful then I can …" or "I wish I was successful so I could … "

You achieve and experience success daily, yes all of you do, and you would benefit from focussing on that feeling, the feeling of success.

As you strive to achieve success, whether it be business, personal, financial or relationship success (these are barometers often used to gauge success but there are others) please remember YOU ARE ALREADY SUCCESSFUL!!! Success isn't or hasn't eluded you …

You are successful!

You have experienced success!

You know what success feels like; it is a feeling within you and it already exists. Focus on its presence and what it actually means to you. What success feels like to YOU.

Recognise, acknowledge and feel the success in your life already.

Success is never lacking. It exists in you now!

---

[1] Lack-based thinking or mentality is thinking based on what we *don't* have. There is a belief that this, in turn, creates more of what we don't have. So striving can often be lack-based as we aren't necessarily stepping forward towards something better; we are focusing on what we *don't* have and trying to get away from it.

Question 67
What is your biggest mistake?

Today's question is not intended to give you another reason to beat yourselves up or dig up old negativity.

It is asked so you realise that however big a mistake seemed at the time, you survived and if you really look at it, you will probably realise you have thrived or at the very least grown as a result of the mistake.

Mistakes can be your greatest gifts!

A life of growth, a life of experiences, a life of worth is actually also a life full of mistakes, of learning. No one is immune to making mistakes. No one!

In answering this question some people have come to realise that what they thought at the time was their greatest mistake actually turned out to be a real gift or one of the major turning points in their life. On reflection I recall someone who realised that what they always thought was their greatest mistake was in fact one of their greatest successes!

Mistakes are valuable and important stages of growth!

Mistakes mean that you tried.
Mistakes are opportunities to learn.
A life without mistakes is a life not being lived.

Question 68
What do you doubt?

This is a powerful, important and interesting question; although I guess not surprisingly, it is often a question people avoid answering when asked.

We don't like admitting our doubts but we are often happy to justify them or listen to them and allow them to silently guide our lives. This frequently occurs without us even realising it.

Acknowledging our doubts brings them out into the open and from there they can't silently, unknowingly guide us.

Facing your own doubts, regardless of their source, means you can question them, confront them and if you decide you can then overcome them, and move beyond them.

A life worth living was never a life constantly directed and stifled by doubt.

Is it time you came out from the shadow of your own doubts?

Everyone has doubts but we don't all choose to listen to them, that is your choice.

"Follow your heart, listen to your inner voice, stop caring what others think."

– **Roy T. Bennett**

Question 69
What do you trust?

An interesting question to explore. I would encourage you to gather as many answers as you can.

Once you have really explored this question then ask yourself, "Do I trust me to be me?"

Fully gloriously you!

What would help you to build and nurture that trust?

When you trust yourself you are free to walk your unique path through life with more clarity and confidence and even love.

The trick to this question, and maybe all of these questions, is trusting your own answers!

"You are powerful, provided you know how powerful you are."

–Yogi Bhajan

Question 70
What don't you trust?

You have been asked two similar but very different questions about trust. What *do* you trust and what *don't* you trust?

Many people answer these questions, especially the 'what do you trust' question, with what they know (or think) they **should** trust.

If you fully trusted yourself and your source (or God, or the universe), you would be living a life of ease. Even challenges would be readily accepted and generally easily overcome.

When faced with these questions, I urge you to go within. To get the benefit of the questions, you must go deeply within. As the questions deepen your commitment and willingness, your preparedness to go within must also deepen.

Don't be tempted to give the 'right' answers. The answers that you think will make you look like you have it all together or you are 'enlightened'.

GET TO KNOW YOU

Does fear overshadow your trust?
Do past experiences affect your trust?
Do other people's expectations or their fears impact your ability to trust?
What don't you trust?

To explore further ask yourself, "Why don't I trust that?"
 Be you, be your truth.

Question 71

What excuse do you use most often?

Often we confuse reasons with excuses or excuses with reasons.

We can become so good at convincing others that our 'excuses' are valid reasons that we sometimes, temporarily at least, convince ourselves:

I don't have enough time.
I'm not good enough.
I'm not smart enough.
I'm too tired.
I can't because of the kids.
I can't afford it.

These are some of my own commonly-used 'reasons' that are actually excuses, I know they can feel like valid reasons at times but the majority of the time they are just excuses.

Excuses can save you from being honest, from admitting something isn't a priority for you right now, or that you just want to say 'no'. Excuses to stay stuck in old, familiar habits. Excuses to not push yourself or risk failure. Excuses to stay in the safety of familiarity however much you think you want to change.

It is common to think reasons are out of our control, whereas excuses can be overcome with our behaviour and actions. This is why we allow ourselves to label so many excuses as reasons; it absolves us of blame and responsibility.

It is time to stop. Stop giving away your own power and incredible potential by labelling your excuses as reasons.

Are your reasons valid reasons or are they excuses disguised?

Question 72
What is your driving or primary intention?

What is your primary intention?

Some people jump easily into this question and others are a little confused, because they struggle to understand the meaning and then to answer it. I invite you to look at it and think about it a little further, a little deeper.

Your intention is important, a powerful influence in fact in what you do, how you do it, what you prioritise and what you ultimately experience in life.

Intention is your aim, your goal, your objective, your plan and we all have an intention for how we live life.

Today you have been asked to focus on your 'primary' intention. Many people will be thinking, *But isn't my intention my intention? What does primary intention even mean?*

When I was first 'gifted' these questions I didn't really understand it and when I asked this is the answer I received:

Your 'driving' or 'primary' intention is often NOT your desired or chosen intention. You have driving or primary intentions and sometimes these differ from your desired or chosen intention.

Your driving intentions can be subconscious and even self-sabotaging. For example you might say your primary intention is 'authentic connection' because is it your desired intention. But if your driving (deep-seated, subconscious) intention is to avoid conflict, you may actually struggle if not find it nearly impossible to be authentic with others. This is because your deep, subconscious, driving intention is actually to avoid conflict above all else. This driving or primary intention will in fact sabotage your authentic connections even though you thought your intention was deep connection. This can leave you confused, frustrated and feeling quite defeated.

Once you are aware of the difference between your primary intentions and your desired intentions you can start to move forward.

So be aware. Do your actions and choices support your desired intention or are you being driven by a deeper, stronger intention that is in fact sabotaging your outcomes and experiences?

Question 73

What or who encourages you to be the best you?

We can all use and benefit from a little encouragement at times. Okay let's face it, sometimes we need a bit more than a little!

How do you best feel encouraged?

Encouragement can make the difference between quitting and keeping going.

Encouragement can help you dig that little bit deeper just when you thought you had nothing left.

Encouragement can help you recognise what you have already achieved and what you are still capable of achieving, boosting your confidence or determination and giving you the fuel to keep going.

When you know who, how, or what encourages you, you can turn to it at pivotal times in your life. You can ensure you surround yourself with it or are at least open to the encouragement.

Surrounding yourself with encouraging or inspirational people, friends, family, colleagues and even coaches, can ensure you have ready access to the encouragement you need right when you need it, maybe even before you know you need it.

It could be a particular person, book, movie, quote or song. Maybe a meditation practice, or journalling or a type of exercise. We are all inspired and encouraged by different things and knowing what or who best encourages and supports us will help us ensure we have the support when we need it.

And remember, don't ever be afraid or reluctant to encourage or support or even inspire someone else!

Question 74
Who do you love?

This question seems so simple and it may be. You may have love all sorted out but for many it is not so simple, not so straightforward and quite honestly not even fun to explore.

Go deeper into this; get below the surface. Explore and sit with your answer. When I first asked myself this question it certainly got me thinking.

What is love?
What does it mean to love?
How does love feel?
What defines love?

I didn't necessarily come up with any definitive answers, but it was interesting to explore, as love is a concept we often just accept and don't really question what does it mean or feel like for me?

That night as I put my then eight year old to bed, I was saying goodnight and I said, "I love you" and she responded with, "I love you too", as she usually does. I then asked her, "What does love mean, what does it mean to you?" She looked at me and said, "Trust and appreciation." Then she got a bit embarrassed and said, "Oh, I don't know."

I said, "I think what you said is perfect. Is that what love feels like to you?"

She said, "Yes. Love makes me feel all safe and I know I love someone when I really appreciate them."

What is love to you?
Who do you really love?

And remember there is no limit to this list; you can never love too many people!

Love, your love, is so uniquely you.

Question 75
What do you love?

You can't consciously choose to do more of what you love until you know what you love. Once you recognise what you love, you can give yourself permission to do it, to build it into your life. You can even schedule it into your day if you need to.

When you do what you love, you are more motivated and that motivation is carried throughout your day.

You will be happier.
You will feel better about yourself and more positive about life.
You will have more fun.
You will even handle challenges with more ease and determination.

Know what you love, what you love to do, see, feel, and give yourself permission to experience more of that!

"One of the greatest regrets in life is being what others would want you to be, rather than being yourself."

– Shannon L. Alder

Question 76
Who do you admire?

It is interesting to explore who you admire and then ask yourself why.

What is it about them?
What qualities do you admire?
Is it who they are, what they do, what they have achieved, or what they have that you admire?
What could you learn from them?

I admire YOU!!

Why? How can I say that when I don't even know you personally?

You committed to a process, you committed to getting to know you, and you are now seventy-six days in. You have committed to showing up each day with faith and honesty. You have made a commitment to nurture possibly the most challenging and complex, and yet valuable relationship you have. The relationship with self!

GET TO KNOW YOU

Here you are at day seventy-six and you are still here, committed to the process and committed to you.

That is admirable!

Question 77

What traits do you respect in others?

Often we respect traits in others that we desire in ourselves, traits that we wish we had.

Can you see any parallels in the traits you respect in others and your own traits?
Can you see areas you could work on or learn from?

Many of us would love to have the traits we respect and admire in others and I believe that is possible. Once you are aware of the traits you admire or respect in others you can nurture those very traits within yourself.

Some common traits people respect are:

Empathy	Inspiration
Honesty	Loyalty
Reliability	Fairness
Positivity	Integrity

Sense of humour	Compassion
Openness	Generosity
Curiosity	Lovingness
Calmness	Commitment
Courage	Politeness

You may see all the traits you admire in one person or more likely you will see different traits you admire in different people.

When you recognise the qualities you admire in others ask yourself, "Do I have these qualities?" My guess is you do and with this awareness you can now choose to nurture them within yourself to become someone you can respect, someone you can admire, someone you are proud to be!

You don't need to change yourself but does this knowledge give you an idea of something you could work on, in yourself? If you admire it in another person maybe you could nurture it in yourself.

Question 78
Who would you like to be like?

It is my hope that this question leads you to an answer that is a version of YOU!

Perhaps a healthier or stronger or more determined version of who you already are, but still a version of who you could be.

When you combine yesterday's and today's answers you will start to get the image of a pretty amazing person. How can you move towards not just being that person but recognising that person in you now? How can you incorporate this into who you see yourself as right now?

You can become a person with the traits you admire, the person you would most like to be, because I believe those traits are within you already. That is why you admire them, why you notice them. You may just surprise yourself with how close you already are to being that person.

What steps can you take now to help bring that person to life, bring them into the light, into your awareness?

Question 79
What do you most like to talk about?

Have a look at your answers. How exciting and positive are the things you mentioned?

The themes are often growth, positivity, opportunity, self, service, improvement, advancement and your own stories and triumphs.

Now ask yourself, "Are the things that I say I like to talk about the focus of the majority of my conversations?" Or do you, like many people, focus on lack, struggle, pain, fear, uncertainty, unfairness, etc. in your conversations? Think about your regular day to day conversations and interactions.

No one ever mentions fear, or struggle or lack when asked this question, yet many conversations revolve around those very things.

Be really honest.

What is your focus?
What do you actually talk about most?

It isn't about being positive and talking about the things you enjoy all of the time, or burying your fears and concerns so you never speak of them; it is about balance.

Work to ensure your scales are tipped in the right direction.

What do you find yourself talking about most?

And never be afraid to talk about YOU! Most of us really love talking about ourselves but we avoid it. This is your life. Don't be afraid to talk about you.

Question 80

What can't you do?

When I first read today's question I thought it was ... well ... stupid to be honest.

"There is nothing you can't do!" screamed in my head. What a limiting, negative belief pattern to reinforce I thought.

I took a breath, okay a few more than one, and I sat with it.

Yes, there are things you can't do, and they can be powerful to recognise, just as powerful in fact as recognising what you can do!

As I contemplated this, I received my answer and still to this day it rings true.

I can't go back to the person I used to be, even if some people might feel more comfortable if I did. I can't grow and stay the same. I can't help everyone and I certainly can't please everyone.

What answer comes up for you?

"Life is too short to waste any amount of time on wondering what other people think about you. In the first place, if they had better things going on in their lives, they wouldn't have the time to sit around and talk about you. What's important to me is not others' opinions of me, but what's important to me is my opinion of myself."

– **C. JoyBell C.**

Question 81
What can't you live without?

How often do you say to yourself or to others, out loud or in your head, "I can't live without … I really need …"

Are you making decisions based on these things you just can't live without when really they aren't necessities at all? What are you sacrificing to have these things?

So many people are working jobs they hate to buy things they don't really need but they think they do.
    Others are staying in relationships that no longer feed their souls because they think they can't live without the person.

What are you doing, sacrificing I should say, to keep things in your life you don't really need?

How much time and energy are you spending chasing things you think you need?

When you get clear on this answer, you will start to realise there is very little you can't do without, and then your awareness shifts and you see you are choosing to do the things you do. Let me say that is fine, we all do it and making choices so you can have certain things is perfectly natural and part of this journey called life. But shifting the feeling from, "I am stuck and have to do this" to "I choose" is very powerful.

Now ask yourself the question again, "What can't I live without?"

Air	Food
Water	Sleep

What else? You will have some others but really the list is fairly short and anything after that is a choice and when you realise you have choices, when you know you are making choices you feel freer.

Question 82
What do you wish you did better?

When you have answered this question I encourage you to delve a little deeper, explore your answer just a little more. Ask yourself:

This 'thing' I wish I did better, do I truly want to do it better or does someone else wish I did it better or think I should do it better?

Do I feel that society thinks I should be better at it or have done better or do I think others judge me when I don't do that 'thing' well?

Do I think I SHOULD do it better?

Is this 'thing' really important to me, or in fact is it not that important and I have just been conditioned to think it is or should be?

Check in with yourself, "Is this really important to me?"

If it is truly important to you, then ask, "What is one step, just one thing I can do to move closer towards being better at that 'thing'? One step to improving myself in that area?"

Just one step, you can do that!

And if you have realised that it actually isn't important to you ask yourself, "Am I willing to let this go and move on to things that are important to me?"

Life is too short to live for other people. Pursue what is important to you. Place value on things that are important to you. Give time to your priorities.

Become the person you want to be.

It is up to you!

Question 83

What does strength look, feel or sound like to you?

Many of us have learned to fear strength and to even avoid appearing too strong. We turn away from it and even condemn it. We judge it harshly. We don't want to be seen as hard or uncaring or bossy.

I was recently asked, "But can I be strong and also kind, considerate and humble?" This amazing lady had been taught and allowed herself to accept, that strength equalled ruthlessness.

When we explored this belief she realised that she had been avoiding being 'strong' as she didn't want to be seen as ruthless, uncaring, hard or unemotional.

Strength is not unemotional; in fact part of strength is knowing you can handle any emotion and being comfortable, or at least willing, to feel all emotions.

It takes strength to forgive.
It takes strength to walk away from situations that don't serve you.
It takes strength to be true to who you are.
It takes strength to ask for help.
It takes strength to pick yourself up after failure or loss.
It takes strength to be true to how you feel.
It takes strength to support others.

Finding your own strength, realising strength is not ruthless or harsh or uncaring and can in fact be loving and accepting, can be truly empowering.

Question 84
What does weakness look, feel or sound like to you?

Do you judge weakness?
Do you avoid it or deny it within yourself?
Do you judge it within others?
Do you do everything you can to hide it?

We all have weaknesses, things we aren't naturally all that good at, things that trigger us, things that touch us deeply.

Do you see these as weaknesses or just parts of who you are?
Parts to be ignored or parts to be aware of?
Do you judge them in others or accept them as part of the greater person?
Do you embrace them or ignore them?
Do you work on them or deny them?

By acknowledging your weaknesses, you can then choose what to do with them. Get as clear as you can on what the weakness is and then ask yourself, "Is this real or am I being overly harsh on myself?"

If you honestly feel it is real ask yourself this, "Can I accept this weakness and allow my other strengths, of which I have many, to shine or do I choose to work on it and maybe over time even turn it into a strength?" If you choose to work on it create a plan, set goals, ask for help and over time, work to improve it!

On the other hand if you decide or accept that this 'weakness' is part of who you are and something you can in fact embrace then you may find that being aware of it and embracing it, allows you to move forward with newfound clarity and acceptance, not just of this weakness but of your many strengths!

The power our weaknesses have over us is often held in the way you look at them. Change how you look at them and the power behind them often shifts as well.

Question 85
Whose voice do you hear in your head?

This question reminds me of a recent experience and subsequent realisation that I had.

Late one afternoon, my husband and I went for a walk. We walked up and around a local headland. I took my camera and was taking photos along the way. We stopped at the top of the headland for quite a while and watched some whales and then watched the sunset.

Three of our kids were at friends' houses and our eight-year-old had stayed at my parents' house while we went for a walk, so there was no hurry, no one to rush home to, very rare for us at the time!

We knew the moon was going to be full that night but we weren't sure what time it would rise. I had left my phone in the car so I couldn't check. We sat at the headland and waited for a while and then decided to leave.

I think my husband said, "Are you ready, do you want to go?" and I just responded, "Sure."

I didn't really think about it too much; I just followed.

As we were driving home over the river we saw the moon; it was beautiful!

In that moment I realised I had wanted to stay at the headland and wait for the moon but I hadn't said anything as I didn't want to 'inconvenience' anyone, I didn't want to 'make' my husband wait. This is such ingrained behaviour that at the time, when we were still on the headland, I didn't even realise I wanted to stay there!

In the car, in that moment as the realisation hit me I knew I had a choice to make, stay quiet or admit what I had done.

For the first time, I said it. I said I had wanted to stay and watch the moon rise but I was so sacred of inconveniencing anyone, including my husband, so scared of being a pain, that I didn't say anything and I admitted that I do this often.

He didn't even question it; he immediately went to the closest beach to see if the moon was still visible. He said he wouldn't have minded staying at the headland if I had just said so.

As I sat after the fact and wondered why I acted like that, why I didn't and often don't value myself enough to be honest about my wants and desires, I realised it wasn't my voice in my own head. It was the voice of my mother, "Keep Dad happy." It was the voice of my teachers, "Be a good girl." It was the voice of random other people saying things like, "Don't rock the boat, don't stand out, go with the flow, don't be a hassle." The list could go on but the reality was it wasn't even my voice. I had taken those voices on as my own. In that moment I realised that I can look back and probably trace it to some childhood events. In fact I know I could, but I decided to release it. I released the belief that I am not worth the hassle, that my desires aren't worth it. I released all of this to the full moon.

I am worth it and I can want whatever the hell I want … whether someone else agrees with me or wants the same things is up to them, but I am entitled to want whatever I want! And if I don't speak up, how on earth can I expect anyone else to know what I want? People, even your partners, are not mind readers and a lot of the time they just trust what you say!

If I don't speak up, even in my own head, how can I know what I want? I have to be the voice in my head.

In that moment at the headland, I didn't even know what I wanted! I actually didn't give it a thought; I just automatically listened to the other voices, the ones I have followed and decided at some point in time were more insightful, more important than my own voice.

It is empowering to realise that no one else's opinion matters more than your own. We must learn to confidently say no one else's measure, opinions or achievements matter more than mine!

GET TO KNOW YOU

I was so thankful for this full moon. Not just its beauty but the lesson it helped teach me.

So whose voice is in your head?
Whose voice do you listen to?

Question 86
What achievement are you most proud of?

Being proud of yourself, acknowledging that feeling of pride, helps build your own self-worth. It helps fill you with a sense of achievement and success. This is a great place from which you can achieve and feel even more success.

Having a sense of pride doesn't have to come from huge successes or public accolades. You don't have to be the best at something or win the race to feel a sense of success and pride.

A feeling of pride can come from waking up with a positive attitude when you have recently fallen into a place of negativity.

It might come from a facing a situation you would normally shy away from.

You may feel it when regardless of the outcome you know you tried your best.

Or perhaps you feel proud of yourself for creating a plan and taking action.

It will be different for everyone. It might come from something big and that is fabulous but it might also come from something seemingly small and that can be just as powerful. The feeling of pride created within you can be the same and it is that feeling of pride, self-pride, that matters, no one else's yardstick or opinion matters!

The size of the prize or the achievement doesn't have to directly relate to how proud you feel of you!

Some days I am just proud of myself for getting out of bed!

Question 87

Do you believe in fairies or magic?

"Who cares?" you might say!

"Maybe no one," I respond but why not consider it and ask yourself the question anyway?

If you do believe, why do you?
If you don't believe, why don't you?
Is it because of what you have been told or taught to believe or is it because of your own experiences and feelings?
Does your answer feel right to you or have you been taught to make it feel right?

One thing I know for a fact is that everything we see isn't real and that everything real can't necessarily be seen. Some of the most powerful things in the world can't be seen.

GET TO KNOW YOU

Did your child-self believe in fairies or magic?
If you did, how did that feel?
Do you remember the feelings, the excitement and expansiveness of those beliefs?

Question 88
What do you dislike about yourself?

Take a deep breath before answering this one.

This is not an excuse to beat yourself up or be overly negative towards yourself; it is about awareness and acknowledgement. We all have things we don't like about ourselves. In fact we sometimes, thanks to our focus, think we have more negative aspects than we really do.

We have deliberately focused a lot on what you like about yourself and you are far enough into this process to now answer this question a little more clearly and to get deeply into what it is you don't like about yourself without over-dramatising it, taking it personally or exaggerating it.

When we shine a light onto the parts of ourselves that we have deemed or judged negative or undesired, or even dark, it starts to take away their power. Nothing is as scary when it is taken out of the shadows and brought into the light.

This may be something you have done. If so what can you do to make amends, to forgive yourself? Denying it doesn't take it away; it just buries it.

One of the things I don't like about myself is that I compare myself to others. Is this something you do? It took this question for me to really acknowledge it. I then asked myself "what is this costing me?" and I realised I was paying a high price. It was holding me back and I wasn't prepared to keep paying that price.

It might be a way you act; acknowledge it and determine if it is serving you, and decide to change it.

It may be a trait of your personality. For example, you may be quick to anger or are judgemental of others. If so, decide if you are happy to live with this or if you want to change it, and ask yourself if you are ready to change it. You can; we have so much capacity to change.

Bring this part of you out into the light and then decide what you are going to do about it. That is empowering!

Question 89
What does God mean to you?

People often say never talk about religion or politics, two subjects that cause division and often emotional and passionate debate and in this book I have touched on both.

Why?

They get us thinking. They make us, if we let them, look deeply at ourselves and our own beliefs and those beliefs form part of who we are. I also hope they encourage you to look at when, how and why those beliefs were formed. I don't want to question or undermine your beliefs, but I do like encouraging you to question and explore or revisit them.

Back to today's question: God

A word that unites.
A word that divides.
A word that offers comfort.
A word that triggers resistance.

A word that triggers passion, one way or the other.
A word that means vastly different things to different people.
A word we can't avoid.

So what does God mean to you?
What does God sound, feel or look like to you?
How does this reference to God make you feel?

Even those who share similar beliefs can have their own personal meaning, feelings and experiences around the word 'God.'

The definition, power and importance of God lies within you and is uniquely yours.

You can replace God with your own word, Allah, Jehovah, Yahweh, Brahman, Goddess, the Universe or many others.

Question 90
What makes you nervous?

Nerves.

We all feel them; they are a fairly universal feeling or emotion.

Some of us take them in our stride and accept them as a part of moving forward, of doing new things, of doing anything we feel passionate about. And there will also be some of us who let nerves stop us, who give them far more power or meaning than they really deserve, who constantly think they are a sign to stop us moving forward.

What do you do when you feel nervous?
Do you mistake nerves for fear and let them stop you time and time again, or do you acknowledge nerves as part of life, especially in new or important situations and proceed in spite of your nerves?

PLEASE know that to feel nervous just makes you human and nerves alone are not reason to stop, to hide, to withdraw, to put your dreams on hold. Nerves are not a sign you are on the wrong path and can in fact be a sign that you are on the right path! Yes, that is right. Sometimes when we are finally doing something that we are truly passionate about, our nerves are at their strongest.

Don't let nerves hold you back; I guarantee everyone feels them. It isn't lack of nerves that sees someone succeed; it is acting in spite of their nerves.

How can you learn to act even when you feel the familiar build-up of nerves?

Question 91
What makes you feel helpless?

What makes you feel helpless?

We often ignore and deny these things. We want to be strong, we don't want to be vulnerable, we don't want to admit to feeling helpless at all so we go on pretending, denying.

Being aware of which situations, experiences or people trigger a feeling of helplessness within you, can help you uncover what is really under those feelings. Knowing what is under your feelings of helplessness can help you realise you aren't in fact helpless!

You may not have complete control or know exactly what to do; you may be uncertain about what decisions to make or how to move forward – but you are rarely truly helpless.

When I explored this question, I started coming up with all sorts of 'expected' answers:

Money	Others' opinions
Illness	Work issues
Death	Our Past

Maybe these have come up for you as you have explored this question; but when I looked more deeply into this, I recognised the following: the only time I feel truly helpless is when I don't listen to my inner knowing, when I'm not connected to me, to self, or when I look outside of me for the answers that are within me.

When I am connected, when I look within, when I follow the next step, I am guided to take and focus on 'the now' and what I can do right now without looking too far ahead. When I am truly authentic I rarely feel helpless!

I feel helpless when I look outside myself, when I forget who I am or that I have my answers within me and when I look too far ahead.

Question 92
What makes you feel capable?

The last three questions are important and if you explore them truthfully, they are truly empowering.

If you can identify what makes you feel nervous, helpless and capable, you will be much closer to identifying your (often) subconscious drivers.

Often our actions, or lack thereof, are based on our feelings, and the feelings of nervousness, helplessness and capability are often behind these.

When we feel nervous, we may mistake it for fear, anxiety or warnings; helplessness can make us doubt our abilities, our potential, our strengths. Feeling capable can push us through these feelings and encourage us to act. Even in the presence of inevitable nerves or doubt.

Being aware of what triggers these feelings within you can help you move past them, act in spite of them or use them to your advantage. And knowing what triggers them can allow you to shift your focus. You can shift your focus from what makes you feel nervous to what makes you feel capable, literally turning a situation around and giving you the push or confidence you need to move forward.

Knowing what 'makes' you feel certain ways is powerful.

If you have been prone to procrastination in the past, these last three questions may be especially powerful for you. If you want to get past your habit of procrastinating or settling, look deeply into what makes you feel nervous, helpless and then importantly capable!

One of my favourite personal mantras I use when I feel scared, nervous, unsure and doubtful is:

I am loved.
I am safe.
I am capable.

What could your personal mantra be?

Question 93
What do you know to be true?

Is everything you have decided to accept as truth actually true?

Some truths serve us, but many don't, and when we explore them we can find that they aren't truths at all; they are just opinions or thoughts that we have played over and over long enough in our minds to make them our accepted truth.

This question is designed to encourage you to question your truths.

Do your truths hold you back or support your growth?
Do your truths encourage or discourage you?
Do the truths you have accepted serve and support you?
As we grow, we change; change is inevitable – does your truth allow for this?
Is your truth expansive or restrictive?
Is your truth an undeniable fact or is it your perception?

Sometimes the truths that drive and direct us are subconscious and we are unaware of them and with this question I really want you to uncover and explore what they are.

Doing this can be so freeing because anything that isn't a definite truth can be changed; you can be freed from its restrictions!

One thing I know to be true is that you are a unique, amazing individual who is capable of so much more than you have yet achieved. Potential surrounds you and is waiting for you to embrace it!

Question 94
What do you believe in?

I believe in possibility and universal abundance. I believe in our ability to overcome any obstacle or past mistake as long as we are willing to move forward and let go.

I believe in the immense power of forgiveness and self-love.

I also believe in self-connection.

I believe self-connection is one of the most powerful and yet overlooked connections we can have. I believe the relationship we have with self is the most sacred relationship we experience.

I believe in YOU!

Yes, I do, I believe in you and your potential and your ability to grow and change and succeed.

But this question is about you. YOU! No one else. You and what you believe in. Not what you have been told to believe in. Not what you have been taught to believe in. Not what you think you should believe in. Not what I believe in.

What do you believe?
What do you believe to be true?
Do you believe in you?

That is where all success and fulfilment begins, with a belief in self.

I hope you believe in you and infinite possibilities because once you do, anything is possible!

Question 95
What do you dream about?

What do you dream about when you sleep and even more importantly what do you dream about when you are awake?

Think daydreams.
Think small dreams.
Think big dreams.
Think wild and crazy dreams.

This question is close to my heart.

When we experienced our 'financial challenge' one of the biggest things for me was that for a while, actually quite a long time, I felt I lost the right to dream. It was almost a greater loss to me than the money!

Dreams felt hopeless and for a long time made me focus more on what I couldn't have, what I couldn't do rather than the possibilities. To dream made me feel angry, hopeless, resentful and a huge failure.

It took me a long time to dream again and not feel like a fraud, not feel like I was setting myself up for further disappointment.

I began by looking around for proof of potential, proof of abundance, proof of success and opportunity. This gave me hope and little sparks of dreams started to take seed again.

Now I dream all the time. It is actually one of my favourite things to do. I like the escape, the possibility. I like trying things out and seeing if they sit with me and my hopes.

Dreaming expands your mind and your vibration past your current reality. Whether you achieve the actual dream is not as important as the expansion that occurs in your energy and therefore in your potential and possibilities when you dream.

And dreaming is fun!

Is it time for you to dream again?

Question 96
What does paradise mean to you?

Paradise   Cloud Nine
Bliss   Nirvana
Heaven   Wonderland
Utopia   Shangri-La

What does this 'place' or 'state' mean to you?
What does it look like?
What does it feel like?
How would you know if you were there, if you were experiencing it?
Is it a place or a feeling?
Is it a state of mind or a way of being?
What is your own version of paradise?

"We are each gifted in a unique and important way. It is our privilege and our adventure to discover our own special light."

– Mary Dunbar

Question 97
Why do you think you are here, at this time, in this place, with the people who surround you?

I believe we are all here for a reason. I don't know that there is a defined, clear path laid out for us to walk, as I also believe in free will, but I do believe you came with an intent, a knowing, a passion or overriding purpose and an incredible amount of possibility. And yes, I believe the timing and circumstances are aligned to give you the necessary opportunities to fulfil a particular, self-chosen, purpose.

Often, though, life gets in the way. Circumstance, drama, trauma, relationships, etc. overshadow your ability to focus on that purpose and if this happens enough, for long enough, you lose conscious awareness of your path. You can lose faith – faith in yourself, in others, in God, in the universe and in your own unique abilities and purpose.

You start doing things to please others, to fit in, to succeed, to get recognition, sometimes even just to survive. You forget to listen to that inner voice, the calling from within that directs you to your purpose. You slip into a type of survival mode and thriving becomes a distance wish as surviving becomes the focus.

Exploring this question, really giving it time and sitting with it, going deeply within to feel the answer can help wake you up to that purpose, the passion, the knowing.

This answer is within you!

No one else has your answer.

Question 98
What are your favourite memories and experiences in your life so far?

Life has ups and downs; that is true for everyone. I don't believe anyone is happy all of the time, but for most of us we desire happiness in our lives. One of the most common answers to the question, "What do you want more of in your life?" is "Happiness!"

At the core of many of our desires is actually a desire to be happy.

I recall some time after our 'financial challenge' I sat down and explored what I really wanted in life. I had been focusing on money and my want and need for more money because I believed at the time it would solve all my problems. After all, the way I was feeling was a result of losing all our money or so I thought at the time.

I sat there in my own bubble of misery and out of nowhere came the words, "I just want to be happy!"

It wasn't about having more money or moving into a better home, or going on holidays, or being able to buy nicer clothes, or going out for dinner. Sure, all of that would have been nice and I had been focusing on it (or the lack of it) for months, but what I realised in that moment was that all I really wanted was to feel happy again. Really happy!

I asked, in desperation, "How do I feel happy when all of this is raging around me and everything is so stressful and I can't afford to do anything fun?"

Happiness is within you, it always has been. Learn to focus on the little things that bring you happiness and your feelings of happiness will grow.

So in the most stressful and challenging time of my life, I decided to shift my focus. I learned and used many tools and I stopped looking outside of me and accepted the answers were within me and change was up to me.

I identified when I had last felt a deep happiness and I focused on and recalled that time. I remembered the events and what was going on in my life, where we lived, how we socialised, and I remembered as much as I could about that time. I did not do this to make myself feel bad about the fact that I wasn't feeling or experiencing it now, but to remind myself that that level of happiness was possible. I had felt it!

I reconnected with that version of me. I learned from her.

I have a photo on my desk to this day taken at that time in my life. Whenever I feel things getting on top of me, or I feel happiness slipping away, I look at it. I look myself in the eye and I reconnect with her and I know that that is possible again. I am reminded of the happiness I felt and that I am capable of that again. I am also reminded how much I want to feel that genuine happiness again and that helps push me.

Life will never be completely smooth sailing; it will have challenges and times you feel anything but happy, but happiness is within you and on your path.

Knowing what triggers those feeling of happiness is a great step towards not just feeling it again, but filling your life with happiness. A step towards happiness.

Really, what is at the core of all we desire?

So often it is a feeling of true happiness. We just want to be happy.

What makes you happy, truly happy?

"Your calling isn't something that somebody can tell you about. It's what you feel. It is the thing that gives you juice. The thing that you are supposed to do. And nobody can tell you what that is. You know it inside yourself."

– **Oprah Winfrey**

Question 99
What negative stories do you tell yourself about yourself, your past, your abilities or your future?

We have all done it and some of us are still doing it - replaying negative stories in our minds, allowing them to guide us from deep within.

These stories may have once been based in truth, but they are past, and we keep them alive within us through the repetition of thought and our focus.

These stories tell us we aren't good enough, aren't loveable, aren't worthy, can't be successful, don't deserve more and in fact sometimes deserve less.

These are just some of the common limiting, negative stories we let play over and over in our minds, quietly directing us, quietly but effectively keeping us where we are, holding us back.

What stories are you telling yourself?
What stories are you listening to?
What stories are holding you back?

What if I told you they are just stories, not truths, just stories and that you have the power and the ability to change them?

You hold the pen to write your own story but first you must stop rereading the old story.

Is it time to create a whole new chapter, be the author of the biggest plot twist in history and write the next chapters exactly how you desire them to be?

Acknowledge the stories you have been listening to, believing and living and then decide what the story, your story, will be from here.

I am handing you the pen, you are the author of your own story.

Question 100
Who are you?

Who are you?

This question is big! This isn't just what you do, or how you perform, or how others see you, but who you are.

As I explored this, I realised that so often we ignore parts of ourselves that we deem unfavourable, undesirable, even negative. But these parts exist; ignoring them doesn't make them go away, and acknowledging them helps us finally acknowledge all of who we are. The whole you!

We are so much more than the titles we carry or the roles we fill. Here I have shared exactly what I wrote when I first completed the Get to Know You process. I am forever changing and growing and evolving just like you are but for now this is me, all of me.

My Real Me

This is the real me!!

I am messy and lazy and hopeless with dates.

I have a jealous side and can be judgemental.

I sometimes think I know the truth and have to remind myself I only know 'my' truth.

I probably don't wash my hair or my jeans enough and if I miss a shower I really don't care.

I rarely go to the doctor; in fact I do what I can to avoid it and I'd rather give birth than go to the dentist!

I hardly go to the hairdresser; I love the result but I hate the process.

I always leave shaving a little too long and I don't get my nails done or have facials and seeing we are being honest I will say that isn't because I don't want to; it is because I don't think I am worth the time or the money.

I don't contact people enough; I think of them often but contact them rarely and even though I am slack, extremely slack, it in no way indicates that I don't care. I care, I care a lot!!

If I write lists, which I could probably benefit from doing, I usually lose them or leave them at home!

I often don't do things 'well' but I do them with love.

I am not great with money.

I hate cooking dinner.

I have fears and I listen to them too often.

I am sensitive, sometimes really sensitive, and I can take to heart what people say and sometimes what they don't say.

I feel responsible, usually for negative things and often for things I couldn't possibly be responsible for. I think you all think 'it' is my fault!

I am all of these things and I usually try to hide these parts of me, to deny these traits. To hide them, however, means denying part of myself and in doing this I often hide all of me; the lines between the traits I desire and those I don't are blurred. What I have realised is all the parts of me are intertwined and in hiding bits of me I hide all of me.

I am more than this though.

I am caring and helpful and loving.

I am a sharer and will often share far more than you expect or perhaps need to know.

I am a giver who loves to help.

I love having a purpose yet I also run from mine!

I am calm in a crisis and perfect to have around when things go astray.

I am considerate.

I am intuitive and when I listen to my intuition, I can be wise.

I can see the world through many people's eyes.

I encourage and support and cheer from the side.

I give great hugs and I accept differences with interest and grace.

I forgive, often even before forgiveness is sought.

I am there without question for those in need, regardless of how much time has passed since we last spoke.

I can feel offended but I try not to hang onto it.

I don't care what others do for a living or have in their bank account.

People are people and all have great value and amazing stories to share and lessons I can learn.

I follow the rules and stress if they are broken.

I am honest and raw.

I am often an open book. If you ask I'll answer honestly, sometimes more honestly than you expected; if you don't ask I will probably stay quiet, or maybe I won't.

I am all of this and more.

I am quiet and loud.

I am funny and serious.

I am the good and the bad, the seemingly positive and negative.

I am the light and the dark.

Remember, without the loud we don't appreciate the quiet; without the dark we can't recognise the light.

At my heart I am a student of life and I am an over-sharer.

I am all of this and together it makes me, the perfect, unique contradiction that I am.

If I deny some parts of me, the parts I deem undesirable, or worse, the parts I think you will find undesirable, and I try to hide them, ignore them, bury them deeper inside, if I do that, the other parts of me can't shine. If I deny parts of me I deny all of me.

This all exists within me.

All of this is me.

I am all of this … and together I am whole.

So who are you?

Question 101

Who do you wish to be?

What can you do right now to become, or move closer to being, exactly who you wish to be?

I am getting closer to being comfortable with who I am but there are some things I would like to add to who I currently identify myself as.

I wish I could confidently say I am:

Successful.
Inspiring.
An author.
A speaker.
That I help many people lead a better, more fulfilled life.
That I am rich in adventure and experiences.
That I am financially secure.

I would love to add these things to who I am and I am working on them.

Who you are, who you accept and allow yourself to be, is a work in progress, it changes, it grows. You have identified and acknowledged who you are in the previous question and in this question, our last question, you get to explore who you would like to be, the things you would like to add to who you already are. We are all growing and evolving. Think about who you would like to grow into and how you would like to evolve.

So, who do you wish to be?
What do you wish to add to the unique you?
It might take time, all change doesn't happen instantly but what would you like to work on?

I can't yet add, "I am inspiring" for example, but I could add, "I can be inspiring." Just take one step at a time.

What can you do right now to move closer to being who you wish to be?

It is up to you!

You create you!! We are all growing and evolving. Think about who you would like to grow into and how you would like to evolve.

Thank You

Thank you for coming on this journey with me. It has been 101 questions; 101 days of self-exploration, and I am fairly confident in saying you have probably never done something like this before.

Even though the 101 questions are finished, this isn't the end of your journey. The journey to get to know and stay connected to self never ends. I have shown you a path, a way to do this, but this is just the beginning. You have laid a strong foundation, but I encourage you to keep building on this.

Some of the questions and your answers would have opened areas for you to explore more deeply, while others may have provided opportunities for growth and change. I encourage you to continue with that self-exploration.

Remember, treat your relationship with self as you would any other valuable relationship in your life; it needs and deserves time and attention. Keep giving yourself time and attention. Getting to know yourself deeper and deeper is not just powerful it is fun!

One of the benefits of this process is you can redo it. As I write this, I have been through the process three times in two years. I continue to be surprised by my answers that change as I change and the deeper insights that come through each time.

How do I know this process works?

I feel it. I know I am connected to me on a much deeper level than ever before. I know so much more about what I want and what is important to me. I am more confident asking for what I want. That doesn't mean I always get what I want but I can finally identify what I want and that for me is a huge step from a few years ago.

On a very simple level, I noticed that if we were trying to decide as a family what to have for dinner in the past, I wouldn't have had an opinion, I wouldn't have really known what I wanted. Now I know. I can easily say, "Well I feel like salmon" or whatever it may be. As I have said, it doesn't always mean I get my way but I am heard.

This book would not have been written and published without me going through this process. You may say *well of course not because the book is the process*, but without going through this process, I would not have become so clear about my dreams or had the courage to pursue them. I would not have had the clarity and confidence to publish this book or any others; believe me I have thought about publishing for over twenty years!!

This process literally changed my life, and I know the impact has been significant on many other people.

I received this feedback from someone who did the first 'Get to Know You' program. She is currently doing the program with me again and when asked question 63 this was her answer:

There have been 2 major turning points in my life. Firstly becoming sober, if I didn't do that I'd be dead. Secondly is when I started following Jodi and did the 'Get to Know You' program for the first time 2 years ago. That program has led me on a continual path of self-improvement and growth. Being sober wasn't enough to change my life. I was sober 4 years before I did the 'Get to Know You' program and those 4 years weren't good at all. I couldn't have done the program drunk but being sober wasn't the thing that changed my life, the 'Get to Know You' program was.

You owe it to yourself to know you. You deserve to have a deep connection with self.

We strive for many things:

Happiness	Relationships
Success	Adventure
Money	Health

But we must know who we are before we can know what we really want, to know why we are chasing what we are chasing, to know what to chase, to have any hope of being on the right path, our own unique path!

So much of what you are striving for starts with your connection to self.

We have all heard about self-love and the importance of it. I struggled with self-love for so long and it wasn't until I created and did this program that I realised why

I struggled. I couldn't love a person I didn't know, even if that person was me. You have to know yourself to love yourself, so getting to know you is the first step in self-love, a step you have now taken.

Never be afraid to put yourself first or take time out for yourself. It is not selfish; it is the foundation of self-love.

Thank you for coming on this journey, for trusting me and for honouring yourself.
Always remember:

Know you
Be you
Love you
Live Life Fulfilled

And never forget you are worth your time. Always honour and nurture your relationship with self. Your relationship with you is the most sacred and powerful relationship you can have.

Much Love
Jodi xxxx

"I finally am seeing the truth of me and I find it beautiful in ways that are conventional and in ways that are not."

"Not everyone will understand or appreciate who and what I am."

"Some wont like the way I look or act."

"Some may even feel fear about things within me they don't understand."

"None of that is my concern."

"The only thing I'm concerned with is finding ways to love and appreciate myself even deeper."

– **Emmie Evolving**